SIRTFOOD DIET FOR BEGINNERS 2021

A step-by-step Guide To Burn Fat Activating Your "Skinny Gene" with Delicious Recipes For Quick and Easy Meals To Lose Weight, Get Lean And Feel Motivated!

Richard Tillcot

Table of Contents

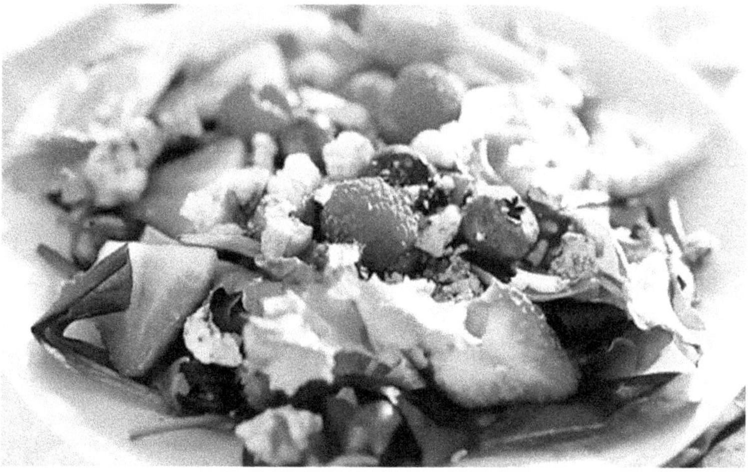

LET'S START!

Introduction

If you've considered taking a diet for weight loss, make sure you have all the truth first.

1) Make sure you eat a well-balanced diet, choose foods high in fiber, and drink eight glasses of water a day.

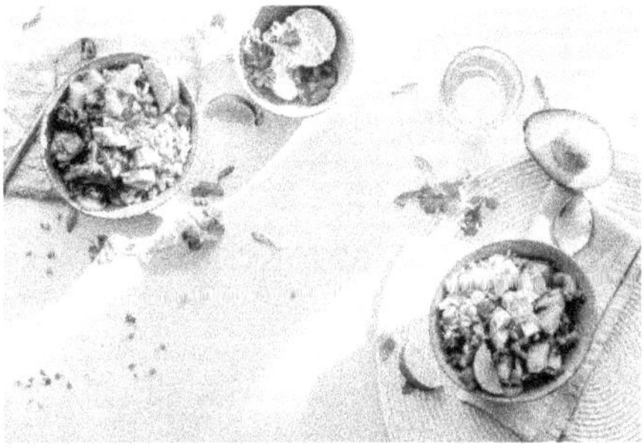

2) Exercise will help lower your blood pressure and the risk of heart disease. Exercise strengthens your lungs, heart, and bones all around. It will keep joints flexible, keep your muscles healthy, give you more energy, reduces stress, anxiety, and depression, and improves balance. That says it all!

3) Retirement, death of a family member or friends, chronic illness, loneliness, and financial stress and concerns can trigger depression. You may need to

be treated with some medication, counseling, or other personal support. Talk to people you can trust.

4) If an accident or spill occurs, it must be diagnosed and handled immediately to prevent any additional ailments.

5) If you are a woman, you should continue to get yearly checkups and let your doctors know all the medications, vitamins, and natural organic remedies that you may be taking.

6) If you smoke, quit - NOW!

7) The best anti-aging cream is sun cream. Limiting sun exposure, using a hat and protective clothing, taking preventive measures to protect your skin, and avoiding sunbeds and tanning salons.

8) The brain functions in the same way as the heart, since blood and oxygen cannot flow through the brain through the arteries, it can't function properly. So avoid fried, artery- clogging foods. Consider

Resveratrol here to address the state of your streets and the strength of your heart if its fast food you consume.

9) Make sure to get your folate intake. Found in artichokes, asparagus, Brussels sprouts, and sunflower seeds, folate is the brain's anti-aging tool.

Another age fighter "in the news" is coenzyme Q10 as it stimulates energy pathways in your brain tissue; and Resveratrol due to its SIRT capabilities. SIRT is a protein

responsible for anti-aging processes such as caloric restriction, alteration of a cells' life span, and an expression of HSF 1, which is another anti-aging factor.

10) Being physically active gives you a much better chance of aging to be more efficient. Determine the types of physical activity best suited for your situation-for instance, if you have arthritis, consider swimming and do it regularly.

The principle of this quick weight loss diet is to eat minimal one day (50 percent of your regular intake) and as much as you like the following day. This process appears to trigger the infamous 'skinny' gene that encourages the body to burn fat.

If you have not come across the diet, here are some of the basic principles:

1. You 'fast' or diet one day, then eat what you like the next day, the next day you go back to the diet and so forth.

2. You should aim to consume below 35% of your regular daily intake on the fasting days if you want to lose weight.

3. The idea is that by having the regular days, once every two days, not only does this trigger the 'skinny gene'; it also helps to trick your metabolism, so that it does not store food.

4. The regular days also help to relieve the usual tedium that can come from regular strict dieting.

5. You should exercise on the normal days and drink plenty of water during the entire diet.

These are just some of the basic principles behind the diet, there are other aspects involved, and the diet includes advice on nutrition and combating the onset of fatigue associated with fast weight loss diets. This mainly involves the correct use of vital vitamins and minerals, as well as a recommended protein intake.

Want to learn more about this fascinating new fast-weight-loss diet breed? Read ON!!!

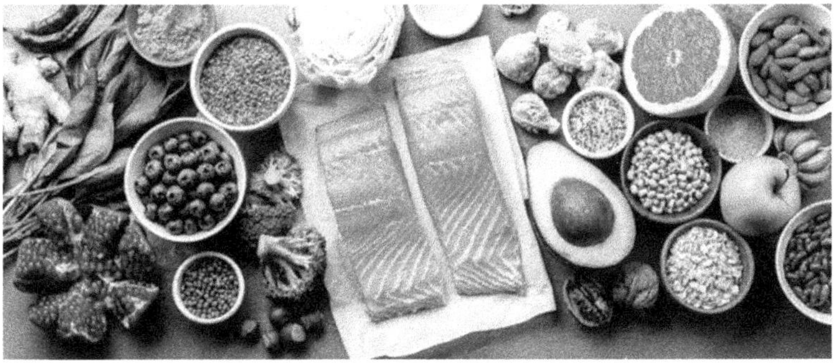

Chapter 1: The Sirtfood Diet?

Such special foods function, according to the creators of the diet, by stimulating different proteins in the body, called sirtuins. Sirtuins are thought to prevent the body's cells from dying while under stress and are thought to control inflammation, metabolism, and aging. Sirtuins are believed to affect the body's ability to lose fat and improve metabolism, resulting in a weight loss of seven pounds a week while retaining the muscle. However, some researchers say this is unlikely to be simply a fat reduction but may reflect improvements in skeletal muscle and liver glycogen stocks instead.

Food

And what are the magic 'sirtfoods'? The most common of the ten include:

- Parsley

- Dark chocolate
- Green tea
- Apples
- Red wine
- Citrus fruits
- Turmeric
- Capers
- Kale
- Blueberries

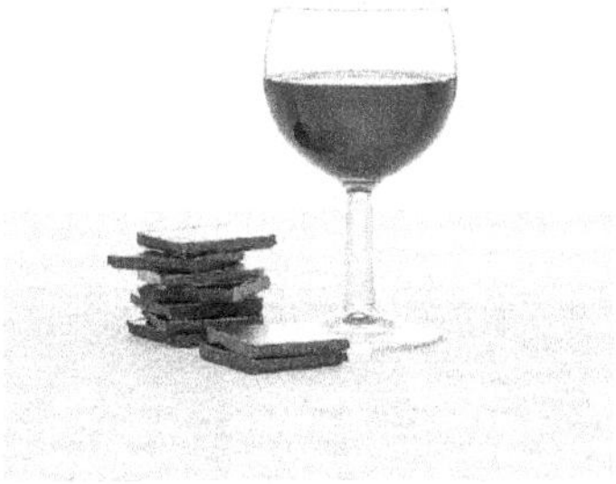

The menu is divided into 2 phases; the initial period lasts one week and includes a three- day reduction in calories to 1000 kcal, intake in three sirtfood green juices, and one meal rich in sirt foods. The juices contain broccoli, celery, rocket, parsley, lemon, and green tea. Meals include turkey escalope with buckwheat noodles, sage, capers and parsley, chicken and kale curry, and prawn stir-fry. Energy intakes from days four to seven are increased to 1500kcal, consisting of two sirtfood green juices and two sirtfood-rich meals a day.

Even though the diet encourages healthier foods, it is limiting, particularly during the initial stages, in both your food choices and daily calories. It also includes consuming water, with the recommended quantities meeting the existing average requirements during step three.

The second period is known as the 14-day recovery process, where there is a gradual weight loss. The writers believe it's a practical and safe way to lose weight. Focusing on weight loss, though, is not what the diet is about – it's supposed to be about consuming the best food that nature has to bring. They recommend three balanced sirtfood-rich meals a day along with one sirtfood-green juice over the long term.

'This is not a diet. I would advise my clients at first glance. It is incredibly ambitious to strive on 1000kcal on three straight days, and I believe that most people will be unable to do this. Looking and understand this piece, you can see that they are the sort of things that frequently appear on a 'healthy food list,' but as part of a more balanced diet, it would be easier to promote them. Occasionally enjoying a glass of red wine or a small amount of chocolate would do us no good-I wouldn't suggest it every day. We should eat a mixture of various fruits and vegetables and not just those on the list as well.

'In order to lose weight and metabolism-boosting, people may have experienced a weight loss of seven pounds on the scales, but this will be fluid in my experience. Burning and losing fat takes time, so this weight loss is incredibly unlikely to be a fat loss. I should be very vigilant of any diet that recommends quick and rapid weight loss because that is obviously not possible and is more than definitely a fluid loss. They will regain weight once people return to their regular eating habits. Slow and gradual weight loss is important, and we need to reduce calories and increase our levels of exercise for this. The harmless way to lose weight is to eat balanced regular meals made up of low GI foods, lean protein, fruit, and vegetables, and keep well hydrated.'

Recipes made with sugar.

These recipes contain foods promoted as part of the diet of Sirtfood.

- Matcha with vanilla
- Turmeric tea
- Date & walnut cinnamon bites
- Red chicory, pear & hazelnut salad
- Italian kale
- Kale with lemon tahini dressing
- Broccoli & kale green soup

- Strawberry, tomato & watercress salad
- Oriental salmon & broccoli traybake
- Superhealthy salmon salad
- Malabar prawns
- Chicken, kale & sprout stir-fry
- Chicken, broccoli & beetroot salad

Chapter 2: Nutritional Value of Kale

The kale vegetable is not so popular among people. It is not widely known. Despite this fact, the kale vegetable can be a healthy addition to many dishes and is worth paying for the next time you shop. If you want to prepare more nutritious meals for your family, then be sure to use kale in some of your prepared dishes.

Kale is a green leafy vegetable that boasts of a mild, earthly flavor. Kales grow well between halfway of the winter and the beginning of spring. This is also the time when the vegetable can be found in abundance in supermarkets, grocery stores, and even outdoor wet markets. This, however, does not mean that the kale is not present all year through. It can be found throughout the year but just in lesser quantities. Another plus to this leafy vegetable is its abundance in most of the year, but it's also very cheap and affordable.

In recent times, the kale vegetable has started gaining the necessary attention that it deserves. Thanks to the advice of most doctors as more of its nutritional value are recognized. And of course, with its high nutritional content, kale is one health-giving vegetable that can be used as an ingredient to many dishes.

Kale is rich in several minerals and vitamins. These include iron, lutein, and calcium for the minerals and vitamins A, C, and K concerning the vitamins. Compared with broccoli, kales have ten times more lutein and an amazing seven times more than the amount of beta-carotene. Kale is also rich in fiber that most people lack in their foods. The vegetable can be a good source of fiber, especially for those who consume many processed foods daily. To add beauty to it is that the kale contains chemicals that protect one from cancer.

These chemicals include sulforaphane, phytochemicals, and indoles. The vegetable also contains the much important vitamin E.

The sulforaphane found in the vegetable kale helps the enzymes that provide the body with detoxification. This helps in the clearing of carcinogenic substances in a timely fashion. The chewing of the kale or the chopping of kale leads to the sulforaphane's production. It instigates the liver to produce enzymes that prevent cancer by detoxifying the chemicals. These are chemicals that we are exposed to daily. Sulforaphane has also shown the ability to reduce the proliferation of breast cancer cells.

The beta-carotene content of kale helps maintain good vision. Vitamin A works hand in hand with beta-carotene to prevent the growth of cataracts. On the other hand, vitamin C is present in the kale and helps reduce the risks of colon cancer.

Kale is presumed to have originated from Asia. It was introduced to Europe by the Celtics. Its importance as a food in Europe was unparalleled, and it has long been the staple food in Rome. The English brought the kale vegetable into the USA in the 17th century.

Kales belong to the same group as the cabbage, Brussels sprouts, and collard greens. This group is known as the brassica. When buying kale, it is important to choose wisely to buy the perfect leafy ingredient for your dishes. Choose kales with leaves that are small in size. That's because the smaller leaves are tenderer and sweeter than broad leavened kales.

Organic Kale Chips

Healthy kale is very nutritious, and many people are interested in how it can be cooked and taste amazing. In this chapter, I am here to share some fascinating details about kale, which will leave you aware and inspired to begin integrating this extremely nutritious green leafy vegetable into your diet for a healthier lifestyle!

Here are some fascinating details pertaining to the kale vine. The best sources of fiber are organic kale and other leafy greens. Green kale produces high chlorophyll levels and is the pigment of plants where photosynthesis occurs. Photosynthesis is the process of the leaves that absorb the sun's energy and transform it into the plant's energy. If we want to consume food with higher amounts of chlorophyll, such as kale, we transfer the solar energy from the kale to our bodies. In effect, this gives us bountiful health and long-lasting strength. Leafy greens, such as organic kale, have a considerable positive impact on the human diet.

This, as well as other green leafy vegetables, are rich in iron and have the highest proportion of phosphorus, calcium, and magnesium. Iron, calcium, and magnesium are all strong alkaline minerals that help detoxify the liver. The minerals bind when our body absorbs these vital minerals to any heavy metals or chemicals stored in the body and then discharged from the body through the urination process.

And now, I'm going to share the most amazing organic kale chip recipe that will make you completely amazed! These kale chips are so tasty that you can hardly resist eating them until you take the first bite! If you have children in your life, making a large batch is smart because they quickly disappear! Here's what it takes you to produce these amazing organic kale chips.

- Four bunches of kale, with a towel, rinsed and patted dry and chopped into pieces of one-inch size.
- Four lumps of olive oil.
- 1 Teaspoon sea salt.
- Two spoonful of yeast for the diet.
- A dehydrating nutrient.

Start by washing your kale under cold water, then using a towel or cloth to pat dry. Then, cut the kale into 1-inch pieces each. Next, put the organic sliced kale in a large bowl and add the olive oil. Now you have to use your hands softly to scrub the oil onto the kale leaves until the wax is evenly covered. Sprinkle the sea salt onto the mixture then rub the kale leaves gently again. The final ingredient is flakes made from dietary yeast. To buy the tasty yeast flakes, you would need to go to a local grocery store. Sprinkle evenly onto the kale leaves with yeast flakes. The final move is to scatter the kale leaf mixture to dehydrate the food at about one hundred and ten degrees. When dehydrated at a lower temperature of one hundred and ten degrees, all of the fresh kale leaves' life-force vitality will stay intact, so do not sacrifice the essential living enzymes of the plant for your safety and nutrition. Dehydrate somewhere between six and eight hours, based on dehydrate capacity. After six hours, check and eat a kale cookie, to see if it's crunchy enough according to your taste.

These organic kale snack chips are so delicious you never want to eat another potato chip! I'm not even joking people here, these chips are the most fun snack I've ever had, and you will never get enough because they're flying too fast! Particularly the children go crazy over them. My kids are constantly telling us to do something, and it's also a perfect way to pass time in the kitchen helping each other make this tasty snack with all the benefits of eating raw organic kale. Please try this recipe and you'll learn snacking in a fun and totally different way healthy way!

Eat Kale Forms and Health Benefits

Today, kale is becoming increasingly popular globally, not just for its fantastic taste but also for its nutritional benefits. While only gaining widespread interest in recent years, many have cultivated and harvested phytonutrient-rich kale for centuries. This freshly minted "superfood" is overflowing with antioxidants, ideal for smoothies, fruits, vegetables, soups, or chip fried. Other leafy greens, like spinach or quiche, can also be used as a stand-in and can be found in soups.

The Kale Popular Varieties

* Kale Curly

Kale Curly is the most prevalent form found in grocery stores and vegetable markets. Why it gets, its name is easy to grasp the top of the green leaves fold over to create a ripple effect. Vibrant green in color, sometimes this leafy variety displays a dark purple running through the leaves. It can have a mildly bitter flavor, but typically only if the leaves are left for a longer time to mature. Kale Curly is perfect for stir-fries and can be steamed or used in soups with lentils.

*Dinosaur (Dino) Kale

Rather than curly in appearance, Dinosaur kale is wrinkled and is more green-blue. With thick stalks and long, narrow leaves, most people claim that Dino kale's taste is somewhat "nutty." You will most often find it in soups, and it is commonly steamed or blanched in hot water or broth. Dino kale is also known at Black kale, Tuscan ale, or Lacinato kale.

*Red Russian

Red Russian kale is quite rare. Red and purplish in appearance, Red Russian has a sweeter taste than the other varieties of kale. Great for making chips, this kale variety is often used as a spinach substitute. Steamed lightly, the frilly leaves make an attractive garnish. If using it in soup, kale should only be added at the end to avoid overcooking.

The wellness benefits kale gives

Kale bears vitamin K, beta-carotene, folic acid, and calcium. It has low saturated fat and low cholesterol content. Kale has also been shown to reduce the risk of at least five different cancer forms. Studies have also shown that kale eating has essential cardiovascular benefits. The kale's high fiber content combines with liver bile acids to reduce cholesterol levels.

So next time you're looking for a great-tasting and healthy new dish to try, give a shot to the kale, and experience all the great health benefits this nutrient-rich vegetable can offer. They're not going to be sorry!

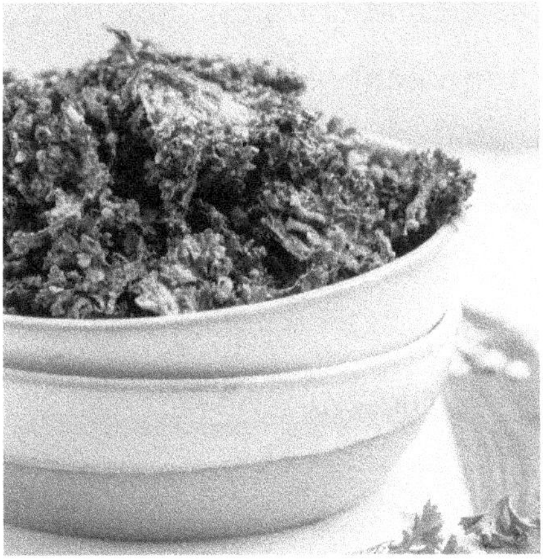

Chapter 3: Onion-A Guide For Creative Cooks

A decent chef knows what ingredients a perfect meal can be mixed to. This piece in the "Ingredients" series focuses on the simple and omnipresent onion. Virtually every kitchen uses the variant onion or onion as a basic flavoring. In reality, Julia Child once said, "It is hard to envision an onion-free world."

There we can take a look at what types of onions are there, their various flavors and characteristics, and the purposes of which onions can be used. When you're done reading, you'll feel even more comfortable going to the store and picking onions, cooking with onions, and making ingredient recipes with onions.

For the onion, the Latin name is Allium cepa. It is related to other edible Allium species: leeks (Allium ampeloprasum or porrum); shallots (Allium ascalonicum); garlic (Allium sativum); and, among others, chives (Allium schoenoprasum). You must immediately recognize those specific characteristics immediately: they all have bulbs, are layered, and taste very strongly. If you're a gardener, you know they 're rising tall and small, there's one flower to one branch, and they're reproducing from the bulb by budding out.

You can note when you reach the store, that there are many varieties of onion available. The popular onions in North America are yellow onion, white onion, and red onion. Small white pearl onions or sweet Walla Walla onions can also be found. Since onions are an essential spice in many parts of the world, humans have cultivated the common garden onion sub-species, also named for their roots. There are various types and uses of these different organisms, and we will discuss those ones below.

On the About.com blog of Peggy Trowbridge, "Sweet Onion Lore," you can find an outstanding guide on the lore of onions in general and sweet onions in particular. The history of the onion is interesting, but not the topic of this post. Here we are more concerned with the collection, storage, and the cooking of onions.

How to place and pick an onion

Onions should be strong and firm, and heavy on the neck. No soft or mushy parts should be in there. The thin skin "parchment" layer should cover the entire onion, but not down through more than one or two thin layers to the nucleus. It's claimed the best onion has 13 rings, so you can't count them at the grocery store.

Onions stay if kept in cold, quiet, dry areas for a very long time. However, once kept dirty, they're vulnerable to being moldy. Do not buy onions with mold on them (the mold can be dry and powdery or, if the onion is very sticky, it can be slime-like algae. If you see mold on an onion, you keep it at home, extract it immediately from other onions and test it for mold. If there is a small mold spot, you should cut it off, so if there is a big mold or the onion is gross, you can dispose of it. Of either in a mound of manure or trash. They are still edible when onions begin to sprout, but they lose some of their flavors. When the sprouts grow big, moisture is sucked from the bulb, and the onion changes texture and taste for the worse. The drier you find them, the less likely they are to sprout.

"Sweet" labeled onions do not preserve as well as other onions and are typically available only seasonally. They are moderate, and taste sweeter than more common onions, as their name suggests. Use these shortly after you have bought them.

Onions come in small sizes as well as huge. I suggest you know how much onion you're going to have at the moment. Buy smaller oignons if you need small amounts of onion to flavor dishes. If you are sauce making and need a lot of onion, go big. Only note that it is difficult to store the cut and peeled onions properly. These will dry out, get moldy, and make the whole refrigerator and/or kitchen smell like an onion when stored in

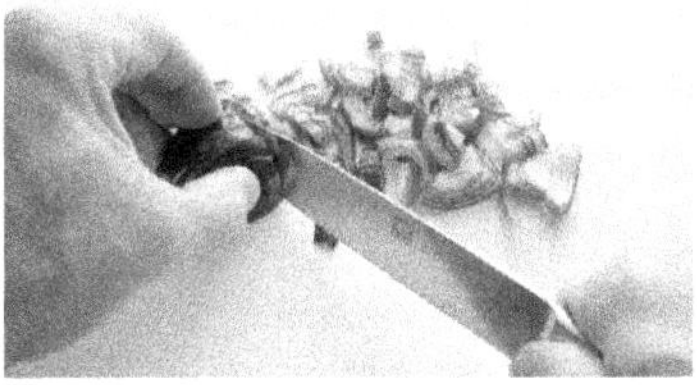

airtight containers. An onion is known as "super-colossal" whether it has a diameter of 4.5" or greater.

The Raw onions

Sweet Onions are the best oignons for eating raw. Sweet Onion varieties are usually only available in April-August, depending on the area in which you live.

Raw onions are often spicy and add a crunchy flavor to cold or hot foods. They can be diced for salads, cut for sandwiches, and pureed for sauces or dressings. They could also be consumed plainly: Russians tend to eat raw white onion with their black rye bread; a popular option is to take a shot of strong vodka, suck in onion and replace it with a piece of bread. (Repeat as required.) Onions could be marinated and pickled in numerous ways too.

It is important to pay attention when using raw onions to the taste and strength of the specific onion you are using. Peeling them under running water will help remove the gases, but using a pair of swimming goggles is the safest way I've seen for really sensitive people. I don't giggle.

How strong is your onion?

While you could buy the same onion brand from the store, over and over again, the taste will be intense and the fumes so powerful that they will burn your eyes, and again they will be mild and almost smoke-free. The intensity of the onion within the same plant varies based on the time of year it is cultivated, the conditions in which it is cultivated, its age at harvest time, how long it has been processed, the consistency of the soil, and the amount of water it gets. When you are cooking, it's important to note and taste the particular onions you've selected for your meal. "A cup of a chopped onion" is just a mass calculation and says nothing about the taste. If you have very strong onions useless, you can use more if they are weak and mild. Even for baking, find recipes as instructions for use in cooking: amounts and proportions are never absolute.

Diverse forms of onions

Yellow Onions make up some 70 percent of supermarket onions. These are easier to grow than red or white onions, have thicker skin, and are not likely to show the green streaks (from the rains of late harvest) or sunburn that white onions may experience. The yellow Onions can be strong or mild, depending on the above factors.

The white onions grow bigger and tenderer than Yellow Onions. They differ a lot in intensity, spice, and emission of fumes like yellow onions. They are very popular with Mexican and Latin American cuisine since they tend to be more tangible and crisper tasting crisper than Yellow Onions. They are very vulnerable to molding, but if kept very dry, they store for a long time.

The red onions grow to a smaller size than the yellow onions. There are even milder and sweeter, with a specific taste and smell. One the variety of red onion is the Bermuda, which typically appears at supermarkets in the spring.

Yellow Granax (sweet onions when grown near Vidalia, called Vidalia), Georgia, and when grown on that island in Hawaii, called Maui Onion). The Cippolini is a sweet oignon from Italy. Other variations include Strawberry Colonial, Carzalia Mild, Oso, Arizona, and Texas 1015Y, a curiously named one. Know these are difficult to store.

Walla Walla Onion (when grown around Walla Walla, Washington), was called Walla Walla Sweets. This onion was born in Corsica and taken by immigrants to Washington.

Pearl Onions, also is known as boiling onions, are small white onions of less than 2 "in diameter. They're hard to peel, but they're a nice addition to soups and stews, and they're a joy to pickle.

Dried onions and Fried Onions preserved

Dry onions are rarely as good as fresh. Just use dried minced onion as a fresh replacement when needed. I stay away from onion powder entirely.

In many Asian food markets, preserved fried (crispy) onions are mostly used to garnish finished dishes, and you can have it ordered.

Cooking in ointments

Onions should only be cooked over medium or lower heat because they change their flavor, and if cooked too hot, they turn bitter. Onions can be cooked in six forms:

1) Getting transparent:

If you cook the onion over low heat for short- to a long time, they will become soft and clear. The more you cook them at this temperature, the smaller they will get and the less noticeable. The approach often used for incorporating onions into sauces and stews is to saute them to clarity. Many sauces start with instructions to 'melt' the onions into some sort of oil, sometimes mixed with garlic and tomatoes. When you place the raw onions in liquid (such as soups and stews) and cook them, the state of clarity is often accomplished. In the first instance, the oil is mixed with the flavor of onions. In the second, the taste of the onion diffuses through the liquid that boils or simmers.

2) Browning:

The flavor of browning onions is delicious too and can be smelled throughout the house (and sometimes even out into the street), particularly when paired with garlic. Golden brown onions are sautéed over medium heat up to the point that light brown color is reached around the edges. When you overcook the onions and roast them, a harsh, salty, burnt taste will replace the smooth, mellow flavor, so keeping a careful eye on the onions is very necessary when you cook them over medium heat. Never cook something larger than average. Green onions are often used as a basis for sauces or stews, but they have not used a very different flavor than transparent ointments. Strong explaining I can offer is they have a toasted flavor. The flavor permeates the oil medium in which it is browned, and so anything cooked in that oil can taste brown onions as well.

3) Fritten:

Unless you dunk the onions in a batter and then drop the hot oil on them, they'll be frying quickly. You need to properly fry onions have a crispy batter and achieve translucent, solid or semi-transparent form. They never have to fire to the ground. Cutting onions (as in Onion Rings) or half of the onion (a common dish in many steak houses) may be fried. For general, fried onions are eaten as garnishes or side dishes.

4) Boiled or grilled:

Onions may be put in an oven and fried, either alone with some sort of sauce (for example, balsamic vinegar and garlic), or as part of a roasted dish (pot roasting, tandoori, roast beef, etc.). Roasted onions can toast thinly on the outside and be crispy in the center, or they can become flat and translucent entirely. The final result depends on how much moisture the platter is cooked in.

5) Freezing:

Grill onions really well but finer to introduce them late to the barbecue grill or skewer because they burn easily at high temperatures. Carefully watch the grilled onions to make sure they brown but don't smoke. Grilled onions don't usually cook long enough to be soft in the middle, so on the outer layers, they are often toasted and soft, and on the inside, they retain some crunch and bite. This makes them a particularly vibrant and tasty accompaniment to heavily flavored dishes such as shishkebob.

6) Marinated or pickled:

Boilers are the most often pickled onions, but if they are sliced, big onions may be pickled too. The best-dressed onions retain freshness and crunch while merging their flavors with strong pickling spices. Most of the pickled onions are boiled slightly (less than three minutes) before they are put in the preservative liquid. This liquid combines vinegar with other spices used in pickling. If you are picking for packaging, make sure that you follow the laws of healthy canning. Pickling is a complicated process, unlike most of the recipes I'm mentioning, and amounts of preserving the liquid need to be weighed with caution. For a great guide, see "Pickle Basics" at Clemson Universities.

Marinated dishes with onions are to be used within one week. The same spices are also used for marinating as for pickling, but the proportions and process are not so significant, because the pickled will not be canned and processed.

In summary, most decent cooks have onions on hand as they are used in many dishes, and onions (non-sweet) are kept for long periods of time. Know how to differentiate the onion varieties by degusting them and using them in your cooking experiments. Out of meager ingredients, a correctly used onion will ring flavor and flavor. When you don't feel like eating, you should only look at the onion. It inspires profound thinking, or at least it influenced the famous American poet Carl Sandburg.

"Life is like an onion: you cut it one layer at a time, and you weep occasionally."

Chapter 4: Benefits Of Turmeric

Benefits of Turmeric

You cannot picture a curry in India without Turmeric in it. Then again, it's just now that people know that turmeric has various superb forces and is much more than a seasoning that can be relegated to a corner on your house. Turmeric is filled with tons of benefits, and nowadays, scientists are further proving this point with science.

Turmeric is a wonder drug that has achieved fame in modern times and has been using it right from medieval times in India. Turmeric is one spice that will typically be found in every Indian kitchen and is used to add flavor to curries and stir-fries. However, its sufficient body is more noteworthy because turmeric is renowned for its anti- inflammatory and germ-killing effects.

Beauticians around the world are waking to the glorious effects of turmeric, and it is now being introduced into beauty goods. What's great about turmeric is that it's readily available, and you can use it in many ways using ingredients that can be found right in your own house.

If you can, otherwise find 100 % pure turmeric powder, you can use it in numerous ways to add shine to your skin.

- Turmeric helps to raise your facial pigmentation and smooth your skin tone. This can be achieved quickly at home. Combine and add small turmeric to the face with cucumber or lemon juice. Hang on for a bit and rinse off. A one-time application may be of little use, and your face would only be given a gentle glow by repeated use.
- Without a pimple? If this is for you or your teenager, turmeric is an element in the beauty that's healthy and still produces strong results. Turmeric, mixed with sandalwood powder and a small amount of water and applied to the skin, will substantially diminish the appearance of

acne. It is, without a doubt, a cheap replacement for all those creams and gels typically not as powerful as desired or they claim.

- Here's a great idea for a body wash all over. Mix gram flour and some turmeric with and water, and use it before your shower to wash all over your body. Doing so sometimes will really help you get a sparkling face. Tell some bride in India, and she'll say this is the beauty regimen that they dutifully stick to days before their wedding ceremony to get a spotless skin.
- One problem that usually besets pregnant women is the physical appearance of stretch marks on their tummy. In case you've wondered exactly how stretch marks can be avoided, consider applying a combination of turmeric with yogurt to the belly, and then it washes immediately after five minutes. If you continue this regularly, it will be surly help in maintaining the elasticity of the skin and avoid stretch marks.

- Turmeric has also been called the super product as a result of its power to attack free radicals. This excellent antioxidant is recognized to help prevent various disorders as well as cancer. Turmeric is one of the best-known remedies used to reduce the restoration time of various skin conditions caused by chickenpox. Turmeric helps even to suppress skin rashes.
- Turmeric comes to the rescue again for those who want to every hair growth on their ears. Regular washing with turmeric dramatically minimizes facial hair growth.
- In India, grandmas also tend to add a turmeric paste to minor scratches, wounds, and bumps because it reduces the swelling much as an ice pack does, without the pain. Turmeric's numerous antiseptic properties are great for using it for minor cuts, injuries, and abrasions, and it assists in quickening the healing process.
- If you have by accident burnt your hand in the kitchen, here's an easy remedy to ease the burn.

Blend a teaspoon of turmeric with some aloe gel and apply it to the burn.

- Up to now, we've studied about the cosmetic results of turmeric for the skin. However, did you know that turmeric is a wonderful natural way to combat that cough that has been bothering you for so many nights? Lose some expectorants, and just blend and drink a spoonful of turmeric with warm milk. The hot milk lightens the throat and the turmeric battle inflammation in the stomach.
- Apply to the infected area about two to three times a day with a mixture of turmeric, rock salt, and mustard oil. Comply with this by rubbing a little warm water in your mouth.
- Felt slow and tired? If you think you have anemia, then a teaspoon of turmeric powder mixed with honey can help alleviate anemia, taken every day.
- Turmeric powder mixed with water is also recognized to help diarrhea.

Just before you get going with some turmeric-related beauty or skin treatments, make a note that it can stain a light yellow face. Using it at night is a good practice, and then washing off in the morning with water and a soft facial cleanser.

As, presumably, you've heard by now, turmeric isn't just good to add to the skin, it also has a host of fantastic benefits after you drink it. It is a fast, powerful spice, without which there is no complete Indian food. As you cook, remember to have it in your meal, and while it may send off a yellow brush, bear in mind all the wonderful benefits you'll receive. The amount of turmeric used in meals is, of course, very small, but it's a healthy dietary practice.

Numerous scientific findings regarding turmeric also reveal that it can prevent leukemia by safeguarding DNA from dangerous toxins. Turmeric also known to minimize the ill results of processed foods and also smoking. Among the active compounds of Turmeric, Curcumin is held responsible for a lot of this benefit.

Turmeric Health Benefits

The highly appreciated Turmeric health benefits come from the rhizomes (root) of this perennial plant found in India. Nevertheless, besides being used for medicine, turmeric does have other skills. Turmeric is a relatively recent addition for most American spice shelves, but for thousands of years it has been a significant aromatic spice in Indian curries. Besides its function as a flavoring spice, turmeric has a long tradition of use in Ayurvedic medicine in India.

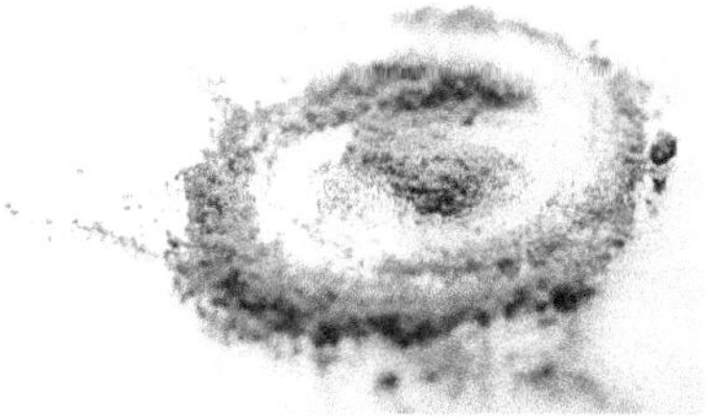

Its presence here is also good news as animal tests indicate that this herb has an amazing variety of medicinal uses. So, let's dive into the turmeric health benefits without further ado.

Firstly, it is important to remember that the chief constituent of turmeric is known as Curcumin. It also contains volatile oils, though, which also harbor medicinal effects.

That being said, let's push on to the health benefits of those herbs.

Turmeric has generated much curiosity in medicine's natural world. This is a strong antioxidant and an anti-inflammatory powerhouse agent. Antioxidants function by neutralizing free radicals, which, if left unchecked, are highly reactive damaging oxygen molecules and can kill cells. Simply put, and antioxidants shield the body from the continuing assault of free radicals that many scientists consider to be unchecked responsible for premature aging and most diseases, including cancer, heart disease, cataracts, and arthritis.

When you have arthritis, perhaps you may be involved in the benefits of turmeric medicine. Do you know that turmeric is widely regarded for its ability to cure arthritis? Turmeric is also used to help relieve pain and inflammation in the arthritis supplements. In fact, test-tube and laboratory tests have confirmed anti-inflammatory and anti- arthritic activity of the turmeric exhibits. Besides arthritis, turmeric may be helpful for other inflammatory disorders such as carpal tunnel syndrome and swelling of the joints.

Many people have specifically a concern in turmeric that has been shown for tumors. Turmeric is currently under investigation for its effects on different forms of cancerous tumors. Several laboratory experiments have shown the anti-cancer efficacy of turmeric. This has been shown in animal studies that the turmeric (curcumin) inhibits various cancers. Evidence from the laboratory results indicates that, according to study, turmeric (curcumin) can inhibit tumor initiation, development, invasion, angiogenesis (growth of new tumor blood vessels), and metastasis (uncontrolled spread).

For example:

- Curcumin (Turmeric) prevented the development of colon tumors.

- Turmeric (Curcumin) has helped stop breast cancer tumor cells from moving to the lungs of mice.

• The growth of prostate cancer on tumor cells in a lab dish has been delayed by turmeric.

Laboratory research facts, meaning animal and laboratory tests, indicate that turmeric (curcumin) has the potential to treat specific types of cancer, including prostate, breast, scalp, and colon. Furthermore, turmeric is known as a cancer-protective herb, as antioxidants help to prevent damage to the cells that begin the cancer stage.

Turmeric health benefits may be of benefit to heart disease prevention. According to a well-known tome written by Michael Murray N.D. "The Pill Book Guide to Herbal Medicines." Statements:

"Curcumin prevents the degradation of LDL cholesterol and damages arteries. Besides, it exerts other atherosclerosis-preventing effects, including lowering cholesterol levels, preventing plaque formation, and inhibiting the formation of clots by inhibiting platelet aggregation.

But wait, there are more turmeric health benefits.

The volatile oils of turmeric are known to have outside antibacterial activity. As such, it may help avoid infections of bacterial wounds.

The herb also stimulates the development of bile, which helps digest fats. In animal research, too, turmeric has been found to have a beneficial effect on the liver, such as protecting the liver from certain toxins.

How is Fibroid Turmeric? We consider scarce details in this respect that the turmeric can be beneficial for uterine fibroids. According to Phyllis A. Balch, the author of the Natural Healing Medication, CNC, Turmeric can be beneficial for uterine fibroids as it is an effective antioxidant that protects the liver while facilitating the removal of uterine fibroidstoxins.

Many potential advantages or applications to turmeric health:

- Indigestion and heartburn can be beneficial.

- It is used to improve the activity of the liver.
- Its antioxidant properties can help to prevent cataracts.

Impact by Using Fibroid Turmeric

The use of turmeric to treat different diseases and disorders dates back thousands of years, and this is an important aspect of ayurvedic medicine. Using turmeric for fibroids, though, is just a recent trend, so you need to hop on it immediately because turmeric has such amazing healing properties.

What's the Turmeric Big deal?

The multiple advantages of turmeric for the skin are nothing new. It's clear that science catches up with the age-old tricks of turmeric, but turmeric research isn't that comprehensive yet.

Turmeric is an incredible spice originating in India and a common feature of Indian cuisine (curries). Spices typically originate from a plant's bark, leaves, roots, nuts, or buds. In this case, the turmeric is obtained from the rhizomes (underground stems) and the roots of the Indian-born Zingiberaceae tree, which is part of the ginger family.

Turmeric is the spice used in the curry to turn it sweet and is part of the black mustard as well.

It's all about one key ingredient.

The age-old secrets to amazing turmeric are the active ingredient that it contains. It is known as Curcumin and has been noted to have very powerful antioxidant and anti- inflammatory properties.

Amazingly, turmeric help with fibroid tumors cannot only support with fibroid tumors, but there are several other disorders for which the use of turmeric as a treatment option entails some benefit;

- Cardiovascular disease
- Diabetes

- Digestive problems
- Alzheimer's disease
- Arthritis
- Cancer
- Liver damage
- Crohn's disease
- Osteoporosis
- Weight loss

In addition to fibroids, whether you're still struggling with either of the above problems, with one stone turmeric kill's two birds, so to speak.

Fibroid Curmeric

Its work on the liver is one of the essential features of turmeric. As described above, it can help in healing and avoiding damage to the liver. For the treatment of natural fibroid, a properly functioning liver is important. Why? For what? Since the liver is an essential organ that helps the body remove waste and toxins. It's necessary to eliminate excess estrogen from the body, too.

Excessive estrogen contributes to a state of estrogen superiority that was responsible not only for the growth of uterine fibroids but also for the rise in tumor size and the occurrence of multiple uterine fibroid symptoms.

Understanding how to regulate the hormone levels and prevent estrogen dominance is an essential feature in both naturally shrinking and preventing fibroids first.

Therefore it is so essential to the liver and why it is so important for turmeric. In addition to avoiding damage to the liver from different causes such as toxins in the bloodstream, it further activates the liver so that it exercises its maximum capacity and eliminates toxins, waste, and pollution. Excessive estrogen can help promote hormone balance and help shrink fibroids and reduce the various uterine fibroid symptoms.

Also to be mentioned is turmeric for fibroids since turmeric stimulates the immune system and helps the immune system better battle against various diseases and conditions, including uterine fibroids.

For natural fibroid therapy such as, you can use turmeric in different ways;

1. Of food and water

You should add the flavor to a normal diet and drink. This can be added to milk, rice, coffee, or some other way that you eat. However, should you want to drink water, try to use a straw to remove the yellow stains on your teeth and use one tablespoon of powder per cup to make sure you drink at least three cups a day?

BUT: The powdered Turmeric sold in most grocery stores that most people use when you drink or use the powder in milk does not contain sufficient quantities of curcumin. Usually, this turmeric contains just around 3 percent of Curcumin, which is insufficient for natural treatment.

You'd need six to eight teaspoons of this store-bought turmeric a day to compare with what you'd find in 1 to 3 Turmeric capsules. This would be impossible to do because you will require at least three meals a day containing large quantities of turmeric, and who has time to do so!

It's also not as good to drink and will stain your teeth. That makes it much simpler and safer to receive the advantages of this main ingredient from capsules. Even if you use the store-bought turmeric and take it this direction, make sure you apply black pepper and improve the body's turmeric absorption, as it can be difficult to digest turmeric.

The body can metabolize this herb easily without applying black pepper, so you won't reap many of the health benefits of this seasoning. Using black pepper can make the body's ability to handle it substantially stronger.

2. Capsules or tinctures

Taking turmeric in the form of a pill or a tablet may be the safest approach because it is less messy and more convenient. Turmeric will stain all of it too. It can take multiple washes to get rid of the stains, meaning you would choose to use turmeric or curcumin capsules to prevent the stains through the use of turmeric spices.

Curcumin capsules are almost as effective if not more effective than raw spice as they contain more concentrated levels of Curcumin, so try either of the above Turmeric or Curcumin capsules for your everyday needs to have a beneficial influence of the turmeric on your fibroid tumors.

If using turmeric for natural diagnosis of uterine fibroids, the generally prescribed dose is around 1,200 milligrams a day, comprising of 400 milligrams of curcumin taken three times a day, or you may obey the manufacturer's recommendations on the capsule label that you want.

A turmeric tincture is another alternative, and three times a day of tinting, you will need around one tablespoon. Drug extract is a tincture. The alcohol is used to remove the herb's maximum benefits and is even being used as a preservative. If you wish to stop alcohol, you can extract it from the tincture by checking online using different tools that you can find.

Caution with Use of Turmeric

These include some of the side effects of turmeric use;

- You can suffer a turmeric allergic reaction that may result in an escalation of the rash or liver enzymes.
- Have a meeting with your doctor if you are using other medicines as turmeric may have a bad reaction to the medicines, so check any medicines you are taking and talk to your doctor first.
- This spice can also raise the likelihood of developing kidney stones in certain persons, as it increases urinary oxalate.

As an important move, you should consider incorporating turmeric for fibroids in your normal fibroid care system, as it is an excellent natural remedy supported by scientific evidence. When you do not yet have a natural fibroid care regimen in place, you will want to find the Fibroids Miracle Guide, which will teach you how to get rid of all forms of fibroids and their effects for good using only natural methods.

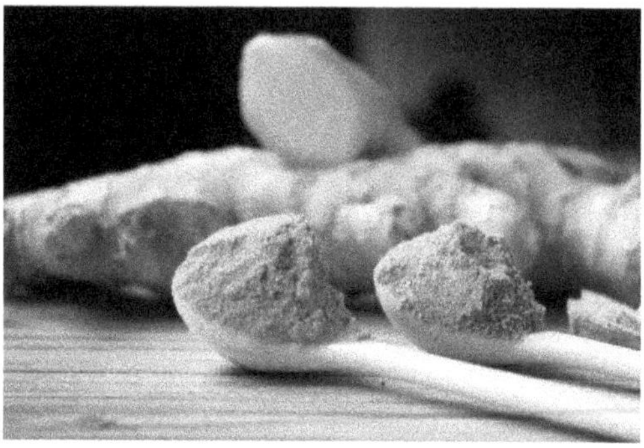

For fibroids, you will have turmeric, but it's just one main ingredient in naturally beating fibroids. The other primary products you need can be included in this natural fibroids care guide that costs less than what you pay a week on breakfast, lunch or dinner, manicure or pedicure, a night out for ladies, etc., and none of those places are useful as this guide.

Chapter 5: Sirt Muesli

If you want to make this in bulk or cook it the night before, just mix the dry ingredients and place them in an airtight container. The next day all you need to do is add the yogurt and strawberries, and it's good to go.

Ingredients:

- 20g buckwheat flakes
- 10g buckwheat puffs
- 15G coconut flakes or desiccated coconut
- 40g Medjool dates, pitted and chopped

- 15G walnuts, chopped

- 10g cocoa nibs

- 100g strawberries, hulled and chopped

- 100g plain Greek yogurt (or vegan alternative, such as soya or coconut yogurt)

Instructions:

Mix all the ingredients mentioned above (leave out the strawberries and yogurt if not served immediately).

Fragrant chicken breast with kale and red onions, chili and tomato salsa

Ingredients:

- 120g skinless, boneless chicken breast

- 2 tsp ground turmeric

- juice of ¼ lemon

- 1 tbsp extra virgin olive oil

- 50g kale, chopped
- 20g red onion, sliced
- 1 tsp chopped fresh ginger
- 50g buckwheat
- For the salsa
- 130g tomato (about 1)

- one bird's eye chili, finely chopped

- 1 tbsp capers, finely chopped 5g parsley, finely chopped

- Juice of ¼ lemon

Instructions:

Then slice it very well, keeping as much of the liquid as possible. Mix the chili peppers, capers, lemon juice and parsley together.

You might put all of this in a mixer, but the outcome is a little different.

Oven to 220OC

/ gas 7.

Marinate the chicken breast in 1 tablespoon of turmeric, the lemon juice, and a touch of oil.

Switch off around 5–10 minutes.

Steam the frying pan oven-proof until it is hot, then add the marinated chicken and cook on each side for about

Then move to the oven for about 8–10 minutes or until light yellow, or until cooked through.

Delete from the oven, cover with foil

But, allow for 5 minutes of rest before feeding.

In the meantime, cook the kale for 5 minutes in a steamer. Fry the red onions and ginger in a little butter, then add the cooked kale and fry for another minute, until soft but not colored. Cook the buckwheat with the remaining turmeric tablespoon, as per packet instructions. Serve with chicken, tomatoes, and salsa.

Sirtfood bites (makes 15-20 bites)

Ingredients:

- Walnuts: 120 g

· 30 grams of dark chocolate (85 percent cocoa solids), broken down into pieces;

· 250 g Dates in Pitted Medjool

· 1 cup powdered cocoa

· 1 tbsp Curcum soil

· 1 tbsp pure olive oil

· one pod of strawberry or 1 tsp of strawberry paste, scraped seed

- 1-2 cups of tea Line-ups:

Put the walnuts and chocolate in a food processor, and grind them until the powder is fine.

Add all the remaining ingredients except water and mix until the mixture forms a ball. Depending on the consistency of the paste, you may or may not have to apply the water - you don't want it to be so wet.

Form the mixture into bite-sized balls using your hands and refrigerate for at least 1 hour in an airtight container before eating them. With some more chocolate or desiccated coconut, you could roll any of the balls to create a different texture if you prefer. They should keep it in your fridge for up to 1 WEEk.

Asian king prawn stir-fry with buckwheat noodles

Ingredients:

· 150G shelled raw king prawns, deveined

· two ts Ingredients-Ingredients:

· 150 g raw King prawns shelled, deveted

· 2 tsp tamari (if you don't avoid gluten, you could use soy sauce)

· 2INGREdients-Components:

· 150 g of raw, shelled, deveted King prawns tamari (you can use soy sauce if you are not avoiding gluten)

· 2INGREDients-Ingredients:

· 150 g raw King prawns shelled, deveted

· 2 tsp tamari (if you don't avoid gluten, you could use soy sauce)

· Extra virgin olive oil 2 tsp.

· Buckwheat noodles (75 g soba)

- 1 Clove of garlic, finely chopped
- Chili of one bird's eye, finely chopped
- 1 tsp, new ginger finely chopped
- 20 g red, sliced onions tsp extra virgin olive oil
- 75g soba (buckwheat noodles)
- 1 garlic clove, finely chopped
- one bird’s eye chili, finely chopped

- 1 tsp finely chopped fresh ginger
- 20g red onions, sliced
- 40g celery, trimmed and sliced
- 75g green beans, chopped
- 50g kale, roughly chopped
- 100ml chicken stock

- 5g lovage or celery leaves

Instructions:

Heat a saucepan over high heat, then cook the prawns for 2–3 minutes in 1 tamari teaspoon and one teaspoon of oil. Place the prawns on a tray. Wipe the pan out with paper from the oven, because you will be using it soon.

Cook the noodles 5–8 minutes in boiling water, or as indicated on the package. Drain and throw up.

Meanwhile, over medium-high heat, fry the garlic, chili, and ginger, red onion, celery, beans, and kale in the remaining oil for 2–3 min. Meanwhile, fry the garlic, chili, and ginger, red onion, celery, beans, and kale over medium-high heat in the remaining oil for 2–3 min. Put the stock on and carry to the boil until the vegetables are soft yet crunchy, then cook for one to two minutes.

Attach the prawns, noodles, and leaves of lovage/celery to the saucepan, then bring back to boil, then extract from the flames and feed.

Strawberry buckwheat tabouleh Ingredients:

- 50g buckwheat

- 1 tbsp ground turmeric

- 80g avocado

- 65g tomato

- 20g red onion

- 25G Medjool dates pitted
- 1 tbsp capers
- 30g parsley
- 100g strawberries, hulled
- 1 tbsp extra virgin olive oil
- juice of ½ lemon
- 30g rocket

Instructions:

Fry the turmeric with the buckwheat, as indicated on the package. Drain one side to cool and leave.

Thinly cut the avocado, basil, red onion, dates, capers, and parsley and mix with the buckwheat.

Break the strawberries, then softly pour with the salad oil than lemon juice. Serve upon a platform rocket.

Chapter 6: Beginning Weight Loss For Health Is Easy

Staying on Track in the Battle of the Bulge

So you have decided to start a weight loss for health programs. That's a great start. Getting motivated to start with weight loss for health can be the easiest part of the process. Maybe you saw an unflattering photo of yourself or an invitation to your high school reunion. Getting motivated, however, is only the first step to successful weight loss for health. Staying motivated is the difference between short-term or yo-yo dieting or success in the long run.

The art of motivational dieting

Committed dieters have learned many tips for keeping themselves motivated over both the weight-loss and maintenance phases of a diet plan:

- Prepare tasty meals. If your weight loss for health program requires you to restrict your caloric intake, make every bite count! Jazz up your menu with spices or exotic flavors. Make mealtime a luxury. With a little effort and planning, you will enjoy your tasty, healthy, and nutritious meal.

- Keep a diet journal. One of the successful tricks of the trade for weight loss for health is keeping a diet journal. Having to write down what you eat each day can give you a sense of pride - or bring to your awareness of your problem eating behaviors. It's been found that people who keep diet journals are twice as successful with dieting as those who don't. You can't argue with those numbers.

- Use a diet coach. You do not need a personal diet coach who comes into your home each day to prepare your meals and coach you to success. The good news is you can achieve similar results by finding someone to help you monitor your progress and offer helpful advice. Some gyms offer diet assistance, as do many diet programs. You can also link with diet coaches online, or use instructional materials available in books and on DVDs prepared by professionals.

Just staying motivated can be difficult for even the most dedicated dieter. Rather than suffer in deprivation or constantly fall off course, look for a weight loss for a health plan that will integrate some of these motivational tools. Find one that provides delicious recipes and meal preparation tips, an organized diet journal, and an online coach who talks with you individually.

Remember that staying motivated in a diet provides the momentum you need to be successful in the long term. Look for a weight loss for a health program that will encourage you to stay on track and provide you with tools you can use.

Diet Motivation Secrets

People are always trying to find a way to lose weight without the pain and suffering of a diet and exercise. Well, sadly, there is no way of losing weight. But the incentive of a person to the diet can be attained.

The diet inspiration is the desire and drives to more regularly consume smaller amounts of healthy foods and exercise. Although doing this isn't an easy feat, some tips and advice on dieting and motivational skills can be used.

You must first determine what your target weight reduction will be to get going on your nutritional inspiration. That's where it gets tricky. Goals have to be realistic and achievable. If we set our weight loss target at 50 kg, yes, it's a great plan for most of us but not realistic.

They'll be useless to our cause because the goals are set too high when they cannot be achieved, so it would be harmful to our food encouragement. Therefore, the goals that we set must be both practical and achievable. It goes with our running ambitions too.

Do not set a goal for 2 hours of work-out per day. That would be terrific to be able to do it, but the average citizen is very incapable of doing it and sticking to it every day. Then you'll raise your standards as you achieve your targets and move up as you go.

The foods that you consume will also need to be changed more than likely. The key to maintaining more weight loss program is that you should expend more energy than your caloric intake. It is that simple.

You don't have to refuse anything you like consuming despite yourself. Simply downsize the servings and feed them in moderation. In reality, statistics suggest that people who deprive themselves of their favorite foods, end up binging on certain foods and leaving their diets altogether.

Also, in the food category, you can get just about whatever you can, but use common sense to eat less, to work-out more to work off the excess you've got.

Diet motivation becomes a habit, just like overeating becomes a habit. Your body is used to the exercises and balanced eating, and after time it becomes normal.

Think positively about obtaining diet motivation. You will feel better, you will look better, and you will have more self-discipline and will power. Those things combined are going to make a better you.

Cabbage Cardiac Broth Diet

The diet for the cabbage soup is also called the core diet for the cabbage soup. Other names; Mayo Clinic Diet, Military Cabbage Soup, Sacred Heart Diet, TJ's Miracle Diet, Russian Peasant Diet, and the Banana Diet are also called. The diet is very popular mostly because it says you can lose 10 pounds in a week if you obey the food schedule. It'll help you get the weight down quickly.

If you're worried about your health, you know that extra weight is a huge concern leading to cardiac failure and blood pressure issues and a whole host of physical problems. But your weight-problems need a long-term solution. Short term diets do not work for weight loss in the long run. By combining exercise with sensible eating, you need to change your lifestyle.

How can the cabbage soup diet work into a balanced eating plan? It's an easy, relatively quick way of falling as much as 10 pounds in a week. The biggest advantage of losing a lot of pounds fast is an inspiration. Many diet plans will only produce about one pound of weight loss per week. That's pretty boring, especially since your normal weight variation can be more than a pound a day. So you can be on the right track to lose weight over the long-term, but the scales show you're gaining weight in the short-term. That's very discouraging. In comes this diet to let you drop some weight fast. Then back, you go to your long-term plan.

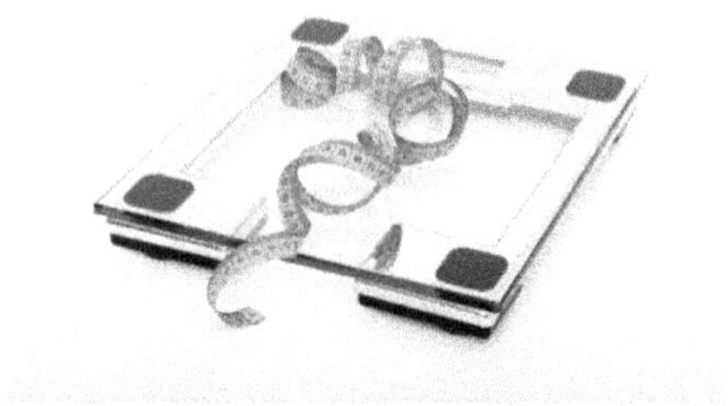

The cabbage soup diet is a great morale booster. And you don't just eat cabbage soup either. You get a set food plan for each of the seven days of the plan. Over the week, you get a variety of foods, including fruits, vegetables, meats, even bananas one day. Plus, all the soup you want each day. And you can vary the soup to suit your tastes. Cabbage soup isn't necessarily bland. You can decide to spice it up as you like.

But alas, no pastries or bread for the week. No brownies, peanut butter cookies, or sweet potato casserole! No sweet desserts. But it wouldn't be a diet without a little hardship would it.

So the cabbage soup heart diet or whatever you choose to call it is a short-term motivational diet to let you drop about ten pounds in a week. It isn't a sustainable long- term plan, but it could be a part of your overall weight loss and fitness plan.

The Basis Diet Programs Atkins eating system

The Atkins diet system is based on the idea that the body is redirected to consume fat instead of carbohydrates to get strength. It's a life-change rather than a diet program because to keep the pounds off, and you need to stick to the recommended eating method.

What you are allowed to eat, i.e., eggs, meat including beef, pork, turkey, chicken, duck, wild game, veal & lamb, including shellfish, is the main difference to other diet programs. The, e.g., butter, olive oil & mayonnaise, and some cheeses are also permitted.

You need to drink plenty of water, taking only de-caffeinated coffee & vitamin supplements like minerals. You also need to work out every day, no need to do a marathon, but a brisk walk will be enough. You are simply encouraged to eat enough to satisfy your appetite, but you shouldn't eat too much.

You will not have to be drinking alcohol. You shouldn't cheat; converting from burning carbs (in the form of glucose) to burning fat takes 2-3 days for the liver, and if you cheat, you're back to day 1.

You can't eat it this way:

Sugar, corn syrup, honey, or maple syrup in any form. Milk or milk-it makes for a small quantity of butter.

Fruit & milk.

Products from the flour (bread, pasta, crackers, etc.) Grains, or grains.

Legumes and beans.

Starchy or vegetables with high sugar such as potatoes, yams, beans, peas, parsnips, beets & carrots.

Sweet condiments like most ketchup, sauce bbq & vinegar balsamic. French styling & covering up thousands of islands.

Cottage cheese, cheese from the farmers & other fresh cheeses. Seeds & Nuts.

Most popular foods are permitted & you can have snacks between meals—no need to starve and are encouraged to eat when hungry.

Diet Program Con's

Must stick to a diet for good to keep off unwanted pounds. No breaks or cheat days you are allowed. If you can't go without a coffee or drink, can isn't necessary.

The South Beach Diet

Related to the Atkins diet system in that it improves the way you eat while also having plenty of traditional foods like beef, fish, and eggs, but you should still consume cheese and vegetables.

You will get three meals a day, plus two snacks a day. You will offer cake & diet soda as well. You are not permitted to drink any alcohol for an initial duration of two weeks, so then you are allowed to drink wine. After an initial two week start where what you can eat is limited, you can start to phase some of your favorite foods back into your diet. It is all about eating "good carbs," rather than "bad carbs."

Pro's food system

Focus on a balanced food strategy, rather than a diet. Much of your favorite foods are still likely permitted. Some alcohol is permitted ie, wine.

Con 's diet program

You can consider the first few weeks, particularly hard since what you can eat is minimal.

The Zone Diet

Developed by Biochemist Barry Sears, The Zone Diet is about regulating the insulin intake by a healthy diet of carbohydrates, proteins and fat, also known as the 40-30-30 diet (40% carbs, 30% proteins, 30% fat). Again, it's not just a three-stage diet to help you lose weight, control appetite & get more strength, and it's a way of life. It is based on stable amounts of insulin, with the inclusion of high-dose fish oil.

The diet in the Zone facilitates feeding consistently during the day and excludes other jink foods such as candy and chips.

The "Area" refers to being in a physiological environment in which hormones are in a region that is not too high or too low, controlled by the food that you consume.

Food program in Pro

A balanced diet rather than cutting out things you ever eat. Con's system of diets

The rationale behind the diet may be very scientific, and many people may, therefore, disagree with its merits.

Mediterranean cuisine

Not a diet as such, but actually a way of living for hundreds or thousands of years, adopted by people from Mediterranean countries like Greece, Southern Italy, portions of North Africa & the Middle East.

Persons from these regions are well known to have a lower prevalence of heart disease; this is thought to be attributed to more than half of their food consumption being monounsaturated food (mainly olive oil), as compared to saturated fat, which is common elsewhere. Saturated fat is known to increase cholesterol concentrations.

The standard diet adopted is one that has low consumption of red meat, medium to moderate consumption of candy, fish, eggs & dairy products except for cheese & natural yogurt, lower consumption of fresh fruits & vegetables & higher consumption of pieces of bread, pasta, rice, potatoes & couscous. Meals are taken with water & red wine (in moderation).

Pro's diet system

A traditional way to eat with known benefits to health but Not a "fad diet."

Con 's diet program

None as usual even if you cannot get new fruit & veg.

Weight Watchers Diet

There are two major diet systems to follow; one is a point structure where all foods are awarded points depending on their calorie, fat, and fiber content. You are required to use a fixed number of points (or use them) every day. The other diet plan is a device of no scores that encourages you to eat from a variety of wholesome foods without counting calories.

Dieting diet plan can be observed online as well as offline by daily local meetings where you can not only provide advice & feedback but fellow weight watchers assistance & motivation.

Pro's food system

You can do anything you want on the points program, as long as you adhere to the number of points. The gatherings can help keep you motivated.

Con 's diet program

Meetings offline may not be realistic for you. The points method will make you feel thirsty.

Chapter 7: Kale

Kale is one of Europe's most prominent leafy vegetables, a wondrous raw food with plenty of redeeming qualities. Really a multinational manufacturer, Kale is used in many popular dishes from Africa, the Netherlands, Ireland, Asia, Brazil, Denmark, the Netherlands, Sweden, Montenegro and Portugal. Despite its incredible health benefits and international allure, kale is still largely under American radar. In Germany, it is so popular, social clubs and festivals have developed around the food, but in America, you seldom see kale being used in restaurants or even in homemade meals. It may bethe temptations of fast food, dairy, baking, and large servings that have left kale mostly undiscovered in the U.S. but hopefully so would the applications of kale as well as fitness and nutrition agendas. No reason why we should not all be cooking with this leafy buddy more often as a super raw food that is relatively cheap and easy to source. Mostly championed and sponsored by fans of vegan, vegetarian, and raw food, each would be best served by having more kale in their everyday eating routines. It should not be challenging for someone to improve their kale consumption, which is very easy to cook with and boast a voracious range of usages. I'm sure there will be a clamor at the stores to buy some after we know a bit more about kale and study its many health benefits.

Kale is a member of the cabbage family and has headless green or purple leaves. Many color combinations may include blacks, yellows, blues, and reds. The vegetable is strong in flavor, and may become even more pronounced after being frozen or exposed to frost. The plant also grows very well in cold and winter climates making it very flexible in cultivation terms. There are many close brothers to kale: Broccoli, cauliflower, cabbage, kohlrabi, rapini, collard greens, and brussels sprouts Kale has many healing qualities and is seen as a superfood. Kale is widely used among its nutritious qualities for garnishing and decoration.

A few Kale Recipes to get you on your way to healthy living! KALE SMOOTHIE (blend well with ingredients):

2 Cups of water filtered in Quatre bananas

Three mangos in yellow 1 Cup of framboise

1 Tassel of red grapes Six to eight Kale Leaves Any Mint Leaves

KALE SOUP (Blend all ingredients to achieve optimal consistency with warm water): 1 Bunch of leaves at Kale

1/4 The Delegate 1/4 Peeled Lemon 1 Tomato di Roma Two cloves Garlic

2 cups of filtered water (lukewarm) A sprinkle of red pepper flakes

Salt, pepper and onion powder to taste

Raw Kale Recipes

Raw kale is one of the most nutritious greens you can eat. Here are three easy raw kale recipes you can try at home.

It is one of the healthiest greens for your bones because it contains vitamin K, manganese, which promotes bone density, and it also contains calcium.

It is also the top green leafy source of the lutein and zeaxanthin antioxidants, which promotes eye health. It also contains C, B6, and B2 vitamins, and is a good source of fibre.

Many varieties are available including Curly, Red Winter and Lacinto. You may also be lucky enough for your local farmer to have an heirloom variety already on the market. Experiment on various tastes and textures of all styles.

There are three simple raw kale recipes here, which I hope will get you to try this very nutritious herb.

Warning: People taking kale are contrain dicatedanticoagulants such as Warfarin.

Tropical Smoothie

- 1 cup pineapple
- 1 cup mango
- One banana
- 6 Latino or Dinosaur Kale leaves
- 2 Pools of vapor
- Make sure you mix all the ingredients in a strong blender like the Vitamix until smooth and fluffy to the complete. If desired, add the honey, agave nectar, stevia or any other sweetener. Enjoy your breakfast routine as a super healthy addition, or as a nutritious daytime snack.
- Green Juice
- Five ribs celery

- One large English cucumber

- 2-3 large Fuji apples
- 1/2 lime
- 6 Curly Kale leaves

Put all the ingredients through a juicer. My favorite juicer because of its The Omega Vert 350 is versatile. If you don't have a juicer, chopping the cucumber, apple, and celery and placing it in a blender (first cucumber) with the chopped kale and peeled lime would be an alternative. Blend this on high for about 30 seconds, then dump over a large bowl and squeeze the mixture through a sprout jar. Sprout bags are relatively cheap and have many uses. The sprouting bag is going to strain all the pulp out and leave you with a smooth , silky juice. Return the juice to the blender carafe and pour it into a glass afterwards.

Raw Marinated Asian Salad

- One large bunch Lacinto or Dinosaur kale thinly sliced
- (or another type of kale)
- Juice from 1 lime (about six tablespoons)
- One tablespoon raw sesame seed oil
- One tablespoon cold-pressed olive oil
- Two tablespoons chickpea miso
- One tablespoon freshly grated ginger
- Two tablespoons finely chopped green onion
- (about two green onions green part only)
- 1 cup finely chopped red bell pepper

- (about 1/2 large bell pepper)
- A handful of your favorites
- [Torn dulse, palm of a silky shore, kombu, wakame ...]
- A spoonful of black or white sesame seeds (optional)

Make sure the greens are thinly sliced, and you can even shred the kale with the slicing disk on your food processor as you wish. Put shredded kale in a large bowl and mash the oil, chickpea miso, shredded ginger and lime juice in with a fork. Making sure the miso is

well mixed with the oil. You can even have your hands massage the kale to make sure the kale is well covered. Serve now, or let the kale marinate for at least one hour in the refrigerator; even it could stay overnight. The longer it gets marinated, the tenderer the kale becomes. Add the bell pepper, seaweed, cucumber, green onion and sesame seeds when you are ready to serve.

I hope you've liked these recipes and I hope you're encouraged at home to eat more kale!

Chapter 8: The Special K Diet Challenge Plan

The Special K Diet Challenge Plan is a diet plan designed around the Special K breakfast cereal, snack, and meal bars. According to Kellogg's Special K website, you can lose up to 6 pounds in two weeks. The average weight loss is five pounds when replacing two regular meals with two Special K cereal meals.

The Special K Diet Challenge Plan is a no-brainer as far as weight-loss programs go:

1. Start your day with any variety of Special K cereal with 2/3 cup of skim milk plus fruit.

2. Replace another meal with another serving of your favorite Special K cereal or Special K protein meal bar.

3. Eat your third meal of the day as you normally do.

4. You're allowed to have two snacks per day, such as fruits and vegetables or any of the Special K line of snack bars, cereal bars, snack bites, and Special K2O Protein Water.

5. Consume beverages as you normally would.

On the Kellogg's Special K website, you can create your own personalized Special K Diet Challenge Plan by answering a few questions with their interactive questionnaire.

I took the questionnaire, and it was pretty straight forward, consisting of just five questions. You answer three questions about your attitude toward dieting and eating habits. Then, you choose your favorite Special K cereal and products for your weight-loss plan. Lastly, you select which day of the week, you would like to start your challenge. The result is a personalized, Special K seven-day diet meal plan. Breakfast, lunch, and two snacks contain Special K cereal and other Special K products, based upon your selections during the questionnaire.

You get to choose your food for dinner.

You can modify any meal or snack by clicking on the individual menu listing and making a new selection from the drop-down menu that appears in the box. You can also toggle between the Week One and Week Two menu plans. You can easily email or print your plan or send it to a friend if you so desire. You're also given the option of printing a coupon for Special K2O Protein Water. You also get special motivating diet tips for each day of the week.

If you don't like The Special K Diet Challenge Plan that you've been given, you can easily reset your challenge and start all over again! Okay, that's the basics of the Special K Diet Challenge Plan. But does it work? And is it healthy?

Pluses:

1. They're going to add calcium to your diet. Yet tests have proven that you can lose weight by taking sufficient calcium intakes.

2. You'll be eating breakfast regularly, which is supposed to help kick-start your metabolism, which also aids in weight loss.

Minuses:

1. There are no exercise recommendations.

2. Nor are there any suggestions for a healthy, non-cereal meal.

3. You'll be getting very little fiber or whole grains.

4. The diet is very repetitive, and you may get bored easily.

In conclusion, the Special K Diet Challenge Plan is very similar to other meal replacement plans. You'll probably lose weight following the plan as you'll be eating fewer calories and less fat than normal. If you want to try a meal-replacement plan, your best bet would be to combine several of them to add a more variety of options.

Diet Journal Advice on Weight Loss Ultra Quick

When it comes to journalizing your diet, putting that into effect and producing a fantastic food journal would help inspire you, making it much easier to lose weight.

Below are potentially considered the top 3 motivational food tips to add to your food diary:

1. Diarise your emotions and thoughts:

This is vital because while it can seem to be somewhat self-absorbing, it is important to be mindful of your feelings because in these emotions is the solution to any issues you may have, and it also makes you understand how you dieted and how you can improve your fast in the long term.

Take, for example, when you're feeling sad or lonely, and at what time in the day, do you consume more food when you have these feelings as your diet plan will reveal.

If so, you need to address these states of emotion and how they can be turned into a positive.

Consider hanging out and catching up with your friends more, or doing something new.

One great place for meeting new folks who have similar interests in your location is meetup.com.

Maybe it's astrology or animals that you have a fond interest in. This is just one website that you can use to your advantage and develop new friendships and advance your interests.

If, however, you feel you may need some professional help, don't be afraid to advise your local medical practitioner.

2. Takedown number of Kg's you've lifted each session:

You should take down the amount in the weight you've lifted each session and the amounts of reps you've completed.

This is vital because you will find that you are now lifting more weights than you were before, meaning your muscle glycogen levels have risen, but you will note that you have not lost any weight.

Do not worry - the reasons for this are two-fold.

a. It means that you've gained leaner muscle mass - you are toning up!

b. A lean muscle mass means you will stay leaner for much longer, making putting on weight that much harder.

3. Take images and print them out:

There's nothing like looking at how you looked a week ago and how you look now.

It may sound like a week won't reflect that much, but only see the little positive changes our body is undergoing.

Make sure you do this from the very start, and it will provide endless inspiration.

Additionally, consider using some of the latest weight loss supplements to help you lose weight faster.

Advantages of Pre-Planning Your Meals

The first important step in healthier eating is pre-planning the meals to ensure a well- balanced and safe diet.

The Strategy Advantages

- Safe options: You have many selections with several different ingredients when you're dreaming about your meal schedule. You should try various types of fruits and vegetables. Also, you should try new, safer recipes.

- Reducing temptations: if you can find substitutes for snack foods with a lower calorie quality, avoiding chips would be easy.

- Enjoyable meals: instead of having regular cereal, create special occasional brunches for yourself and treat yourself differently. I'm looking forward to having the food and doubling the enjoyment you 're receiving from the meal.

- Monitoring progress: it will also be easier to make a clearer evaluation of your diet schedule with a smartphone workout program or by holding a weight loss log. You'll be able to check your success by keeping track of the meals from the previous day.

- Nutrition schedule: if you plan a day's food in advance, you'll be able to take better care of your wellbeing. Your days will also be full and filled with events, and you'll find it better to plan a nutritious meal in advance.

Ideas to add when it comes to eating out.

- Safe snacking: When you dine outside, your diet schedule can get affected. Whether you are bringing crackers or a bag of nuts along, you will end up ordering lighter, because you will always feel loaded.

- Call for ahead: review your menu options before booking a seat. Check that custom orders are being made by the kitchen and whether they have calorie counts on their menus.

- According to various research, things that eat have a big effect on the calories who consume. Order in a group first, so that you can influence others.

Ideas to apply at home

- Smart Shopping: try filling your shopping cart with freshly produced goods instead of putting in processed foods when you go shopping at grocery stores. The foodstuffs that hit your kitchen should be safe to your core, and nice to your waistline.

- Arranging the food: the first thing you can see is safe when you're starving and going to the kitchen; otherwise, you'll have to eat more. Hold it tucked away and out of reach when you're in the kitchen for some fast food where you'll just feel lazier to find it.

- Cook immediately: if you keep yourself concentrated on make-ahead dinners, you'll feed your children more than you do.

- Measuring parts: The component sizes will be identifiable and common to you.

Preplanning meals will help keep your weight stable and provide you a positive eating par. While it is not easy to consume and sustain a safe lifestyle with balanced diets, the effort is worth it that you put into it. A proper diet does not only ensure health, but it also makes you happier. The suggestions we mentioned above help you make choices about what you can eat. If you're eating outdoors at a friend's or a bar, these tips will help you know whether to eat and keep your lifestyle safe without compromising on all the fun and socializing.

Chapter 9: Recipes For Coffee

A coffee diet! I've heard the lot now. The second thing you know, with tea and cookies, we'll be making something like 'lose 10 pounds in 7 days!!' I mean, who comes up with these fat blasting ideas? Or, more importantly, who buys into them? You can imagine it in the staffroom at your workplace. Everyone fighting to get their Cornish pasty in the microwave, and there's you quietly preparing lunch with nothing but a kettle. Okay, ribbing aside, I guess we should look at this diet in a little more detail and see what method is behind this seeming madness.

Anyway, moving on a tad, the advocates of the coffee diet propose that anyone who wants to shed a bit of weight should do the same as my mother's suggested. However, they did not refer to her; you understand!

However, this weird weight loss approach needs to be looked into a little deeper before we all jump onto the coffee diet bandwagon mouth first. I say, there's just an array of get- thin-quick ideas going around these days, it's wise to take a few steps back to take this situation into account. That refers to all of the latest fads and not the caffeine diet alone.

It is best to first pay a visit to a own doctor before embarking on some new weight loss plant. A complete physical never hurt anyone, and your physician will have valuable insight into the coffee diet approach. Still, somehow I can't see any responsible doc giving the thumbs up to drinks for food diet. Take the coffee diet to an authorized nutritionist, and I bet the response is the same. I could be wrong, though, and through these two visits, a coffee diet is probably the right thing for your weight loss needs.

You know, we're always looking for the next lazy, or should I say easy, no, perhaps effortless weight loss program, but despite it all, the old fashion way still wins every time. Can you remember the original diet? It's merely to put less in your mouth and get more exercise. That's it! Okay, so there are a few whistles and bells to add like the right types of food and a sensible exercise regime, but you get the idea.

Another factor worth finding out about the coffee diet is that it is simply a fast cure and not a fresh way to eat (or starve), and maybe if the dieter sees that as a kick start to a more rational food schedule, it's not so bad. It also went on to say in the article that the coffee diet is not the foundation of the program. Now, this probably doesn't make a lot of sense, so I'll try to explain. Advocates of the coffee diet strongly urge you to eat well throughout the day. By well this, they mean to adopt a healthy food diet consuming small portions as part of the regime.

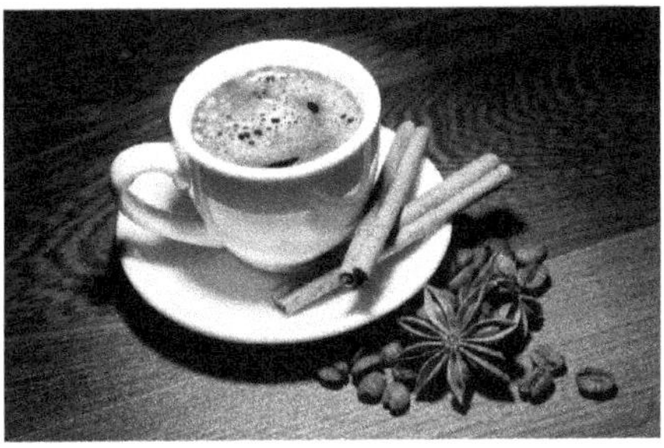

The coffee diet allows the dieter a moderate intake of coffee throughout the day, but the coffee has to be pure. Lattes and cappuccinos and all those other fandangled coffee cups are out. Hmm! It sounds okay, but at the end of the day, we're still not eating properly because the coffee diet is removing our natural appetite, and I'm not convinced that's a good thing.

One final point that may give you food for thought is your insulin. Caffeine can make your blood sugar unstable. The insulin in your body will not be able to process it properly, and it winds up stored in the body as fat. So, if your decision to take on the coffee diet, make sure that you don't drink too much.

People make drinks for coffee in several different ways. If you're going to make your coffee at home, you may want to do it exactly this way. For you, here are two simple coffee recipes: cappuccino and granita.

Cappuccino sauce

The cappuccino was first prepared in 19th-century Viennese cafés. It received its name from the words "capuchin friars," which is the color of the local monks' robes.

Services 2

Products-Ingredients:

2 Express, short servings 1 Cup of milk

Disposal:

- Pour the milk into a saucepan
- Put the espresso maker's steam nozzle a third of the way into the pitcher to make the milk foamy, and open the steam valve all the way.

- Do not let the milk boil or get too hot. Put the thermometer for the candy into the pitcher. Heat the milk to 175 degrees F. Evite heating the milk too hot. Close the Valve for steam.

- Have espresso packed. Pour into serving cups until roughly a quarter of the cup is filled with coffee.

- Stir the milk into the serving cups before pouring in. If you've poured much of the milk into the coffee, place a spoon under the milk, you're pouring on top of the coffee to create a coating of foamy milk.

- Willing to serve.

Recipe by Granita

A granita is a semi-frozen form of coffee. Its usual ingredients include Includes caffeine, coffee, and tea.

Services 4

Products-Ingredients:

6 Espresso servings, at room temperature, short 3 Spoonfuls of sugar

16 Cubble of ice 2 Cups hot water Disposal:

- Pour espresso in a blender. Stir in the water.
- Add 90 seconds of sugar and espresso together. Stop the Mixer.
- Add ice and water to taste. Mix in until smooth.
- Pour into cups to serve.
- Willing to serve.

Look for more Recipes for Free Coffee?

Greek & Turkish Recipes

There are many people who know how to make Turkish coffee in a simple cup but Turkish & Greek Recettes

Many people know how to make a simple cup of Turkish coffee, but some not-so- traditional Turkish and Greek coffee recipes:

Greek "Ouzo" Formula Caffee

This is a popular Greek monk coffee recipe in the sacred "Agio Oros" You need to: 2 Greek coffee tablecloths

2 Sugar Teaspoons

1 "ouzo" teaspoon (typical Greek alcohol) Water: 2 * 3 oz cups

Add the Ouzo inside after you have prepared your coffee, and serve. By "Koniak"

This is a popular Greek Seamen coffee recipe. It's the same as the previous recipe, with the only difference that you use Koniak instead of Ouzo.

With "Honey"

This is an old Greek coffee recipe from Smirni. Prepare your Greek-Turkish coffee, and then add one teaspoon of honey. It's delicious!

With "Cardamom"

This is a sort of Arabic version for the Turkish coffee recipe. Use a dark coffee blend ground for Turkish. Get some cardamon, and grind it or use a mortar. Two seeds per cup are enough.

Cardamon is used to spice up and give an aroma to the coffee. You will need: Two teaspoonfuls of coffee

- 1-2 teaspoons of sugar as much cardamon as you want
- 2*3oz cups water

- Prepare coffee as usual. You will get a delicious exotic coffee, which is very different from anything you've tasted before! With "Mastich"

- Same as the above recipe but instead of cardamom you must use mastich (only produced in Chios island, Greece)

- Turkish Coffee Recipe with "Fennel Seeds"

Same as the above recipe, but instead of cardamom, you must use fennel seeds. So, go ahead and enjoy great coffee!

Spanish Coffee Type Recipes

My recipe here will concentrate on Coffee Recipes "Spanish" style. If you like Spanish cuisine, I think that you would like my recipes for coffee too. Then, wait.

Classical Spanish Recipe for Coffee

You learn how to make coffee latte of a "Spanish" kind from this recipe.

Materials

Appropriate for one human (High glass)

1) 4 cups of Spanish coffee syrup

2) 1 Bio espresso shot

3) 0.75 teaspoons of low fat steamed milk Fittings Desired

Electronic blender and espresso maker Preparation Steps:

1. Take the blender cup clean and empty, pour all of your ingredients into the cup. Mix it for a bit, before it mixes equally.

2. Upon completion, take a large empty bottle and pour the hot coffee into the container.

3. Finally, now you can enjoy your Spanish Coffee.

Spanish And Latte Coffee Recipes

Another type of cold Spanish coffee drink for those who like cold beverages. Materials

Appropriate for one human (High glass)

1. Spanish coffee syrup and chocolate syrup two tablespoons, respectively

2. 1 Vegan espresso shot

3. 0.75 Cup of steamed low-fat milk

4. 5 to 8 cubes of ice

5. Some whipped cream (optional: you can put some whipped cream if you like it)

Pieces of Equipment Needed

Espresso maker and electronic blender Steps for preparation:

1. Take one blender cup and put all of the ingredients into the cup except whipped cream, which will be using later.

2. If you like cold coffee, you can now put some ice cubes before you blend it.

3. Blend it with low speed until all well mixed.

4. Take an empty glass to pour your latte into the glass.

5. Finally, if you like whipped cream, put it on top of the latte before you serve it.

Mistakes In Creating a Healthy Coffee Recipe

Coffee is one of these days' most popular beverages because it contains anti-oxidants. Not to mention, coffee provides other health benefits as well. However, several individuals are beginning to search for a safe coffee recipe from which they can make use. Sadly, some persons make errors in doing so. To stay clear this, below are some of the errors that individuals will be conscious of when making a safe recipe for coffee.

Think all oil is created equal

One of the principal choices for making a balanced coffee is to add oil. The error made by individuals, however, is that they believe all the oil is produced equal. For starters, adding coconut oil to a coffee will offer wonderful health benefits. It is not safe to use ordinary oil; however, as the benefits provided by raw and unrefined coconut oil can be overlooked by using ordinary ones. The easiest thing to do is make sure you pick the right oil for your recipe.

Choosing the sort of butter you are using

The next error individuals make in making a recipe for coffee is that they ignore the sort of butter that they use. Butter is an important ingredient for making a good coffee, as is oil. This is possible because butter can provide burnt fat to become energy. Still, this can only be done by using grass-fed milk. Worse still, some people use margarine that is considered to be a hydrogenated fast fat.

Stir in milk

Certain people would, of course, like to make their coffee tasty. And adding milk, is the best choice. Surely, milk can have great health benefits, but it will kill its good characteristics by adding it to your cocktail. This effect is felt as milk can constrain the body from the fat-burning role that balanced coffee can offer.

Requires sugar

Adding sugar is also a huge mistake that individuals make when it comes to making your beverage sweet.

Sugar is something of a carbohydrate. Hence the skeleton will burn carbohydrates and store the fat, which can defeat the purpose of the drink rather than fats. In case you want to make your drink sweet, it is best to make use of natural sweeteners.

Using ordinary coffee

And then, some people make use of ordinary coffee, too. Most coffee is contaminated with pesticides. Individuals thus consume those chemicals that can affect their health. Fortunately, some companies offer organic coffee beans. To prevent pollution, these beans are packaged in natural containers.

These are all just a few of the mistakes individuals make when they create their healthy recipe for coffee.

Nowadays, more and more people know how important is a healthy body is to us. People are now looking for foods that are good to us, especially on low-fat, low-sugar, and low- carbohydrate foods. Today, coffee recipes are specially designed for people who like less sweet coffee to respond to this group of people.

First Coffee Recipe: Low Sugar Peaches and Spice Latte Recipe

If you are looking for something that contained low sugar, this recipe is especially so for you to enjoy a cup of low sugar latte.

Ingredients

Enough for one person

1) 2 tablespoons of peach with low sugar and cinnamon syrup respectively

2) 1 Bio espresso shot

3) 0.75 tablespoons of low fat steamed milk

4) 3 or 4 cubes of ice

5) 1 small spoonful of cinnamon powder as a garnish to use at the last stage

Equipment Needed

Espresso maker and electronic blender

Steps for preparation:

1. put together all the ingredients in the blender cup except garnish, which we will use later.

2. Blend it with medium speed for 1 minute until they are well mixed.

3. Take an empty glass to pour your latte into the glass.

4. At last, Spread the powder of cinnamon top of the latte before you serve your latte.

Second Recipe: Low Sugar Raspberries and Spice Latte Recipe

Another low sugar coffee recipe that I specially created for the coffee lover that likes to consume very little sugar.

Ingredients

Enough for one person

1) 2 tablespoons of low sugar of Raspberries and cinnamon syrup respectively

2) 1 shot of organic espresso

3) 1 small tablespoon of Cinnamon powder as garnish

4) 0.75 tablespoons of low fat steamed milk

5) 1 to 5 cubes of ice

Equipment Needed

Espresso maker and electronic blender

Steps for preparation:

1. Firstly, you need an empty blender cup for you to put syrups, espresso, steamed milk, and ice cubes.

2. Blend it for 60 seconds until they are evenly mixed.

3. Take a tall empty glass when finished, to spill your latte into the bottle.

4. Cover the cinnamon powder over the latte, before serving the friend.

Chapter 10: Staying On The Diet

We all know dieting can be a heck of a challenge, especially if you are not used to eating healthy or if you have poor eating habits, start with. Yet it certainly must not be an impossible feat.

One of the greatest errors so everyone makes is that they come at the wrong perspective at dieting. A "diet" is nothing to be considered or frowned at as a short-term fad. This should not be perceived as something that you are using for a "fast remedy" to a weight issue or safety condition. A diet would be a comprehensive lifestyle change, in a way, a thorough redesign of your eating habits. Your food is meant to become your way of life, a method of eating that you hold to for the long haul on a regular basis.

This should make it easy for you to be inspired and stick with it when you start talking about your diet this way.

Start Little

The first idea of having yourself on a diet is choosing to change your eating habits for the better. You'll need to give yourself a long-term dieting target. Say you want to become a full-fledged 100 percent vegetarian or vegan, for example, or you might want to eat only organic eventually. The very easiest way to get you started on your path towards reaching your target is to continue with tiny, practical improvements.

You won't become a vegetarian or vegan immediately, so if you're planning to achieve so, you're more definitely gearing up for a disappointment. Changing your diet is like changing any other habit you may have, and time, effort, and motivation will be needed. Motivation should be the secret to being effective on a diet.

Taking Baby Steps Diary

Now that you've settled on your long-term objective of dieting, the next move is to chart how you can do it. You want this plan to be mapped out one step at a time. Of starters, if your aim is to become a vegan, you can start by replacing a one-day meal with a "vegan meal." Alternatively, you can do something like having a single weekday, your "vegan day." Reasonably and wisely, choose your baby steps. It's certainly clear you can tell more about yourself better than anyone else, so you can make up your mind to start with either one meal or a whole day.

Stay Motivated

The best part of taking one-on-one baby steps is that this is what will help you stay motivated on your new diet plan. The trick to continuing on the path to dieting progress is to make practical improvements, one step at a time. Each time you take one of these baby steps, you'll feel proud of yourself, which will keep you inspired to keep going on and sticking to your diet schedule.

When you back up, meal by meal, or day by day, your baby steps slowly turn into leaps and boundaries. Before you know it, you should be well on your way to reaching your dieting target. It will be simpler and safer to stay motivated with every action you take toward your goal. The new lifestyle will become a "force of habit" when you get to the final phase of the plan.

Never again fail a diet and exercise program

Why will too many diets and exercise plans fail to send in? What causes the rate to be so alarming? Was the system to blame?

Obesity is mounting at an alarming rate. Lots of people are experiencing major changes in lifestyle. Food routines are bought paying for Gym memberships, but after a few hours, and all diet and fitness plans have been discarded! Sure, the gym pass may not have been revoked yet, because they say that they will start exercising again soon, maybe!

And what's going wrong exactly?

Why are so many people quitting early? This lets people think it's just not worth dieting because they're destined to fail. One of the biggest causes, why diets fail, is that people want to see progress, 'Soon.' They're almost hoping to miss a few meals and 'Hey Presto' as if by chance all the weight is going to be gone miraculously.

People have grown to expect instant outcomes, maybe a magic pill. The question is that miracle pills aren't available anymore. Unable to see a diet out to its end will make the diet struggle worse; most people add the extra pounds on.

MOTIVATION & common sense are essential to producing efficiency. You've got to get the right attitude for the enduring inspiration. Adequate strategy, the will power.

Once you know this and first work on your motivation issues, you are more likely to reach your goals, and your health and fitness lifestyle will be in the past. Deep inside, you have the motivation in you. You may. You may. Your family or friends may be helping you, cheering you on. This will help increase your motivation.

When you hear of people failing with their diets and exercise programs, they realize that it is not the program that is failing them. They are wrong. We have declined to demonstrate their inspiration.

Motivation to Break The Course

Your enthusiasm will most likely be the determining factor in your diet. You must remain focused, determined, and motivated until the end. Having support from family, employers, and experts will help keep you focused, but eventually changing your lifestyle is up to you.

If you're overweight or clinically obese and want to shed weight, you've got to take responsibility and stick to 'The Plan.' Eat the right diet, don't snack, and follow a good routine of practice. You'll need a decent 8 hours of sleep every day, too.

Seek to keep your thoughts concentrated on the intended outcome. Believe in Himself. Trust, you should. Trust that. Think about the outcomes, and how you feel when you reach your goal. Then, your attempts don't seem as intense. If you start thinking like this, it will be easier to remain motivated and focused on your goals. Become the guy you really wanted to be. Succeed on your diet, and you'll eventually find that you're hoping for a more positive conclusion. A person who knows that what they started was they should finish. They will make it to their targets.

Choose the right diet and exercise program to suit you.

Do not only leap blindfolded into a diet system. Make sure the right program is chosen, as this will give you a huge advantage in achieving your goals.

The health and fitness sector has become saturated with programs to lose weight, some good, some bad. The reason for this is that so many people lack the determination and fail miserably only to blame the program. They then continue to the next diet plan hoping for a 'Quick Cure,' and yes, the same thing is happening. People end up consuming diet plan after diet plan without the correct attitude and the continued inspiration. The diet industry won't let you inside their secret. We don't want you to know it's you who lack the drive, the desire to achieve, the appetite, the inspiration. Yeah, it's a rough walk, but it's worth it. You know it. The problem is that the food industry needs to market foods, and they continue to promote foods. Hundreds and thousands of pounds are expended, and if you're not patient, you'll end up in this relentless, vicious cycle that's sure to make you add even more weight!

Finding a diet and exercise plan which suits you can get complicated. Researching for a viable diet program that will help you achieve your weight loss and fitness goals, as there are so many available, can take time.

There's so many admitted 'experts' out there who would drive you to diet items they don't recognize. They know that if they sell it, they will get a fee!

One of the easiest things to do is make sure you research just what sort of diet it is, and do the fitness routine that matches you.

You need to get sound advice from a doctor if you have any health problems or are obese. He'll be able to propose a plan that won't just be good for you but safe to follow!

Maybe the local library will help. They have dieting and fitness books in their racks, and if you take my advice, if it's close enough that you can, you'll walk to the library. This will be a good exercise for you.

Research online, as well as offline, will give you a good idea of what to expect from a diet and workout plan.

Remember, don't let them scare you and remain motivated.

Forums online are a perfect place to be. You will converse with like-minded people and get the help you need to thrive. People will even clarify what diets they've tried and maybe propose one. But be careful. Some of the people there are not after weight loss, and they're just there to peddle diet books they're affiliated with! So be warned, do your homework and keep on watch. Don't actually follow the first person's opinion that you communicate with. Make a note, and further investigate the product, if possible.

Using each program you are studying, try to figure out just what it takes to accomplish your goals. Think about what you're going to have to do, how much time you 're going to have to spend, whether you're able to do what's expected of you, what equipment you 're going to be expected to use, what kind of outcomes you 're going to expect and how soon you can achieve success. Knowing this will help you agree about the correct food and fitness schedule. Another that has a greater chance of succeeding; what you need to do is add yourself, inspiration, and determination. Talking to a professional person will help lead you in the right way, but again, don't let their excitement push you in the wrong direction. The diet and fitness regimen can be fantastic, but if it includes things you don't like and workouts you simply can't do, it would be pointless to you. Before you commence, you are doomed. Research, research, and then have a good idea about all of the benefits and minuses of the program before making your final choice.

It's fast!

Don't jump into and overdo the current fitness plan. You are likely to end up in pain or worse, and you may be hurting yourself. You need to get off to a slow pace. 'Take it easy' and slowly work your way up over a few days or a few weeks.

As your exercise levels rise along with your confidence, you'll soon be able to complete a full workout. If necessary, take advice from the Gym staff. They're the talkers. They are qualified to advise well, so take care.

The best approach is to work your way up to any level. Maybe you should start your first day with a brisk 20 to 30-minute walk. You should add five minutes to that each week before you hit the target of 1 hour. Having started at a level that's too difficult will leave you to believe you can't achieve it, that you can't reach one's goals. You'll give up soon. And make no mistake in overdoing it.

This is true for your diet too. Don't give up your favorite foods at once, as this may depress you and cause huge cravings for unhealthy food. Depression will also hamper your weight loss strategy when you're stressed, and the body releases a cortisol hormone. This hormone is known as the pain hormone, which is likely to disrupt the mind and body. That hormone could well dampen your excitement, and faster, you'll be helping to give up your dream.

You might continue by treating yourself with a couple of the unhealthy foods you enjoy eating right now. Then give up one gradually per week until you end up with just the remaining balanced diet. Even if you eat a perfectly rigorous diet, you should still treat yourself with one meal you enjoy every week. We want to call it a gourmet dinner. It's your treat, your reward for holding on with your diet, and you'll be offered everything to look forward to.

You have to ease back into a current long-term exercise routine, so you shouldn't start all at once abruptly. Start slowly, then develop momentum continuously. When time goes on, your body should be able to adjust to the harder workouts and conform to the smaller size portions that your diet demands.

Just don't plan to lose weight from the places you like. Slowly and evenly, you will most likely lose fat from all over your body. Many people are under the impression that concentrating their work out on a certain part of their body would allow all the weight to come off that 'Spot.'

I've seen males do hundreds of crunches, working day after day on their 'Six Pack.' Hour after hour, hoping they'll end up with a well-sculpted 'Six Pack.' Not so, you can crunch none for 24 hours a day, and it just won't happen. It's not until you get your body fat down to around 10 percent or less. Try to tell them, and they won't listen.

Make sure that you realize this and simply focus on other techniques that will help to burn the fat quicker. Unless you want your swimwear to look healthy, you'll need to concentrate on losing the fat and developing lean muscle. Dieting without exercise can help you lose weight, so it's getting rid of both lean muscle and fat. The only problem with that is that you'll continue piling weight on if you stop dieting. All that weight is fat and not muscular. And you just lose healthy lean muscle to replace it with fat!

Concentrating on different parts of your body every day can be a good thing. This will allow you to work out various parts of your body that have not had a great deal of exercise for a few days. It will allow parts of your body to rest while you continue to work out another part of your body!

It's easy to work overtime yourself and find that the next day you can barely walk. This will cause you to quit the gym. Take it slow and avoid the issue. Realize that this is not the fault of the program; it is the way that you have chosen to approach it.

Friends and Family

Keeping motivated is the best way to make sure you stick to your chosen fitness program. The best way to do that than getting a family member or a friend to join the gym and also to follow your fitness program.

Failing that, at the gymnasium, you will make friends. This way, because they have been a regular for a long time before, your new buddy is still working out at the gym and far more likely to keep going. That will increase your motivation and help you focus on your exercise program even more.

You are more likely to feel bored and disillusioned if you cannot exercise on your own. Although working with friends is going to promote some friendly rivalry. See who will shed the most weight and keep each other accountable. You do not want to let down your girlfriend, and you will find that you are looking forward to exercising with your friend / s.

Start your diet program, and tell your mates.

Try your diet plan and get your friends involved. Build curiosity in a Buzz, and they'll help drive you towards your target. Don't stress if your mates at first want to be teasing you. It will always support you as long as you, in the right way, bear their ridicule. Using their bullying to build within you a roaring fire which makes you want to prove them wrong. Your mates can keep you going even though they don't know they do.

You'll find that while you're around your friends, you're going to put off eating the wrong food and want to impress them with your diet any further.

Friends will be a great aid when committing to a fitness plan. They help build a feeling inside of you that makes you want to stick in the health system even though they don't talk.

Measuring Great

Keep track of your results and how you've made progress, as this helps keep you highly motivated. Even if the results are minimal, you'll find that you're one step closer to achieving goals set and becoming the person you want to be.

Measure yourself at workout start. Weigh yourself and do your BMI job out. How far can you go before you lash out? This will keep you updated on how you profit from your new lifestyle.

When you can measure your food and fitness program advantages, it can excite and inspire you. You won't see the score every week. It speeds down as time progresses, and you lose weight and gradually look as if the weight loss has come to a standstill.

Give yourself a reward, and it will help you keep focused and on track. Nutritious snacks should be better to treat. If it's a walking trip, which involves any sort of exercise, you might reward yourself with a trip after you've lost some weight.

Do not treat yourself with food. It could be disastrous, and people often think of food when a treat is mentioned—unhealthy food treats. You have to distance yourself from unhealthy food as far as possible and try to stop thinking about it.

Looking at a new mirror, you'll have motivated you soon, and you'll be able to congratulate yourself on that. Taking pictures can allow you to see how you interpret various stages of your diet. Perhaps you will know you are well on the way to achieving your goals.

A fresh, smaller outfit, and perhaps a pair of jeans, will be needed soon. This holds the energy all on track. You’re going to want to strive ever more towards meeting your goals soon. Only say you don't press too hard. Note, build steadily upon the pace.

You'll have days of course where you feel a bit sad, 'you can't move on!' It is here where your inspiration should kick in. Get off the treadmill to use inspiration to inspire, inspire yourself!

Most people don't stop practicing in the gym because it's too hard; they're quitting because they just don't want to go to the gym. They could not get upset. Skip off one day, and skip another one. Don't. Do not. Drag yourself down to the gym to complete these sets of workouts. Once you're in there, you'll feel better. A lifelong habit you've got to break. Consider it your workout routine.

You'll find that if you drag yourself down to the gym, you'll likely end up with d = completing a full workout, and you'll feel better inside. "Go on. Could you do it!"

Failure of fitness plan

Most people believe the fitness routine they are pursuing isn't going to work. We fear they won't maybe produce the results they desire. If you let them, these thoughts will quickly get you to give up your goals. You have to adopt a positive approach to your exercise program. Keep your mind focused on all the advantages the fitness routine has to offer. Giving up now will make abandoning next time easier. You are going to find yourself criticizing the program, not yourself. Do not go down this route; otherwise, you will be trapped in the illusion that these systems are not effective.

Think of the advantages. The sexier body, healthy heart, and improve physical fitness. That will help you stay motivated to the end.

You'll find that you'll have more faith in a better one, and you'll start feeling less sluggish. You'll find you can spend more quality time with the people you're around. Will, you do not want to see your kids grow up? Even play a greater part in their lives and even the lives of their children (Your grandchildren).

That all comes down to your motivation and perseverance. You want to live a healthier life. You want to look the best you can. You want to be a little mobile.

DO NOT GIVE UP. STAY FOCUSED. STAY MOTIVATED

ACHIEVE YOUR GOALS NOBODY CAN STOP YOU. ONLY YOU!!

Join your food and fitness routine for as long as you can, and let it become your way of life. Fight for health and fitness. Fight until you can't go on until there's no fight left. Make what you once thought was impossible, and take it even further.

It'll amaze your family and friends. Some might even be somewhat jealous and wish they had the Grit and Determination to achieve their goals.

The New You is waiting for YOU...

You'll know your diet doesn't have to be too strict, and you don't have to kill yourself by pursuing an exercise program. Allow your life better and view your diet and exercise as your daily way of life. A lifestyle you like to adopt, something you're proud of.

Weight Loss Menus

How often have you attempted the latest generic fad weight-loss menus promising to the world yet leaving you frustrated, exhausted, and still struggling with your weight? Well, read on to find out why these fad diets don't work, and what you can do to boost your weight loss chances of success.

1) First of all, you're an individual, and the way your body responds to food is different from the next person's. It is partially due to the body shape and metabolism. We each have the opportunity to eliminate weight and tone up; we just need to know what works for our body, and not for someone else.

That's why some people can lose weight on "one-size-fits- all" diets, but most are still left disappointed. If you don't deal with your body and its desires, you'll be chasing your tail and irritated by your lack of progress.

2) More often than not, the food set in concrete for you to eat is boring, tasteless, and nutritionally deficient. If it's not the right type of food for your metabolism or given in the right combinations, you're not going to get very far.

3) No variety. The biggest reason people struggle at diets is that they get bored with tight eating regimens and lack energy. Diet programs need to be full of a range of products, and versatile to change for you as the expectations for weight loss change.

4) The fad weight-loss menus are more often than not full of hard-to-find or costly food items, further hampering your inspiration. Weight reduction meals need to contain readily available or conveniently substituted items from the nearest grocery store.

5) They sometimes recommend guidelines on unhealthy diets. Some don't encourage eating fat, and others don't encourage carbohydrates and high protein. Everybody completely ignores the fact that you are a person, and eating this way for your sort of body will cause nutritional deficiencies and make you feel flat and exhausted. Essential carbohydrates and fatty acids are essential to a healthy body. If you deprive your body of them on one of these fad diets, your body becomes malnourished, causing a host of unpleasant symptoms to develop.

I encourage you to study the fad diet books and look into having your weight loss menus tailor-designed for your body size and condition to meet your weight loss goals.

Conclusion

In conclusion, the sirtfood diet is focused on the premise that certain foods in your body cause sirtuins, which are particular proteins believed to reap different benefits, from shielding cells in your body from infection to reverse aging. Green tea, dark chocolate, bananas, citrus fruits, parsley, turmeric, broccoli, blueberries, capers, and red wine are all items included on the menu.

Proponents explain on the official sirtfood diet website that there are two "easy" phases to the diet. Stage one is seven days with three sirtfood green juices each day and one sirtfood-filled meal — a total of 1,000 calories. Yet don't be discouraged: On days four through seven, you may feel marginally less hungry if you are allowed to raise your intake to 1,500 calories with two green juices and two meals. Phew, yeah!

Phase two doesn't look much more promising. This process lasts two weeks, during which, in addition to your one particular green juice, you are required to have three "healthy" sirtfood-rich meals per day. The goal is to encourage more weight loss during this period. While the sirtuins' benefits seem promising, the sirtfood diet is being marketed as yet another way of "Losing seven pounds in seven days!" You know that drastic diets don't work like that by now.

Here are three things to take bypass with the sirtfood diet:

From a weight-loss perspective, the sirtfood diet only tests a success.

I've said it before, and I'll repeat it: Weight is a determinant of health, but it's not the only one. Measuring someone's health success on whether they're losing X pounds in X amount of time ignores all of the other food benefits. Meat is full of nutrients, and you can do stuff like showering, exercising, and breathing. It also has nutrients that can facilitate multiple body functions and is also a historically based enjoyable activity. There's much more to focus on for better quality of life than just size, and it's un-useful to determine outcomes only in terms of weight loss.

It is restrictive and can harm your food relationship.

This diet stresses a daily intake of between 1,000 and 1,500 calories, which is much smaller than most people need. When our food intake is severely limited, our instinctive reaction is to overeat. Your body is wise and views this lack of sustenance as an assault. Hence we appear to overcompensate, which is why we can all contribute to being "hangry" and then overindulging until we have a chance to eat. It is a more natural way to exercise healthy and intuitive feeding than to limit calories.

The sirtfood diet isn't based on science.

Although there is some controversial study on the benefits of sirtuins, there is little to no research on the specific diet for Sirt foods. We have some standards currently in place that have been carefully studied and checked for decades. When you're lost on what "good eating" is, that's a great starting point.

If you want to integrate a few sirtfoods into an eating plan, it's okay. Foods such as green tea, bananas, dark chocolate, and kale each have a place in a balanced diet after all! Adhering to a system that has such stringent pass-or-fail requirements is impractical and may be harmful to your relationship with food. You would be able to develop a long-term, healthy relationship with food by implementing an eating schedule that is full of variety and eating attentively. Cheers to it!

Lightning Source UK Ltd.
Milton Keynes UK
UKHW021844040521
383144UK00003B/384

9 781802 743340